Palliative Care in Emergency Medicine

What Do I Do Now?: Emergency Medicine

SERIES EDITOR-IN-CHIEF

Catherine A. Marco, MD, FACEP
Professor, Emergency Medicine & Surgery
Wright State University Boonshoft School of Medicine
Dayton, Ohio

Palliative Care in Emergency Medicine

Edited by
Tammie E. Quest, MD

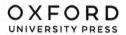

OXFORD
UNIVERSITY PRESS

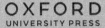

Oxford University Press is a department of the University of Oxford. It furthers
the University's objective of excellence in research, scholarship, and education
by publishing worldwide. Oxford is a registered trade mark of Oxford University
Press in the UK and certain other countries.

Published in the United States of America by Oxford University Press
198 Madison Avenue, New York, NY 10016, United States of America.

Library of Congress Cataloging-in-Publication Data
Names: Quest, Tammie E., editor.
Title: Palliative care in emergency medicine / [edited by] Tammie E. Quest.
Other titles: What do I do now?: Emergency medicine.
Description: New York, NY : Oxford University Press, [2023] |
Series: What do i do now?: Emergency medicine |
Includes bibliographical references and index.
Identifiers: LCCN 2022040662 (print) | LCCN 2022040663 (ebook) |
ISBN 9780190073824 (paperback) | ISBN 9780190073848 (epub) |
ISBN 9780190073855 (online)
Subjects: MESH: Palliative Care | Emergencies | Case Reports
Classification: LCC R726.8 (print) | LCC R726.8 (ebook) | NLM WB 310 |
DDC 616.02/9—dc23/eng/20221206
LC record available at https://lccn.loc.gov/2022040662
LC ebook record available at https://lccn.loc.gov/2022040663

DOI: 10.1093/med/9780190073824.001.0001

Printed by Marquis Book Printing, Canada

Contents

Preface

Palliative care in the emergency department? What is that? This question is often asked among emergency department colleagues and peers—much less so now than in the past. While it has been nearly two decades since palliative care in the emergency department setting became a focus of study and organized implementation of optimal palliative care delivery, emergency clinicians have always faced caring for patients of all ages with serious, life-threatening, and advanced illness in the emergency department. It was not until the evolution of the practice of hospital-based palliative care that a real appreciation developed by those within and outside of the emergency department, setting the real and potential impact that providers in the emergency department with optimized palliative care knowledge and skill might have on the care of patients with serious illness. Over these two decades, the emergency department–specific and wider palliative care literature has burgeoned to demonstrate improved models of palliative care within and outside of the emergency department with a concomitant burgeoning evidence base. This evidence curve will continue to evolve with care in the emergency department increasingly as a focus. Over the last decade, study after study now has shown that patients who receive palliative care in the emergency setting with and without a palliative care subspecialty consultant have improved clinical outcomes with better symptom management, improved goal concordant care, and more effective resource utilization that delivers improved patient-centered outcomes. Palliative care is now widely known as the physical, spiritual, psychological, and social care provided from diagnosis to death or cure of a life-threatening illness provided at any stage of illness and *in any setting*. Palliative care in the emergency department is fundamentally meeting a seriously ill patient and family wherever they are, be it in pain or in cardiac arrest, and providing the best care possible—not only focused on disease reversal. Palliative care in the emergency setting is the clinician formulating a multidimensional assessment that includes mitigation of suffering and distress in all its forms. For some patients that might require not just an assessment of what can be done but what should be done based on the patient and families' goals and values. Sometimes this might include breaking bad news or helping mitigate severe breathlessness while also treating sepsis and much more. The lynchpin to effective palliative care in the emergency department is the emergency clinician.

Palliative Care in Emergency Medicine is intended to serve as a practical resource to the emergency clinicians on the frontlines of emergency care. Imperative to the practicing emergency clinician in delivering palliative care in the emergency setting in a practical way is to understand it in breadth, concept, and practice. While not exhaustive as a textbook, this book will cover a wide variety of critical areas in palliative care in the emergency setting in a format that the clinician can easily grasp and follow: case discussion. Each chapter is authored by an emergency clinician, often paired with a palliative medicine subspecialist to consider care options. In many cases, the author is both an emergency clinician and palliative medicine subspecialist. Each chapter opens with a typical emergency department clinical case that any emergency department clinician across the globe might be asked to manage, followed by a discussion, conclusion, and suggested readings. The discussion is meant to focus on the practical aspects of working in emergency care that is often punctuated by incomplete information and stressors felt by the patient, the family, and the clinician. The suggested readings represent key articles that inform the discussion and encourage the reader to go further in depth on the topic at hand. Some key areas explored through case discussion format include an overarching understanding of emergency department palliative care; critical communications; advance care planning; symptom management; care for special populations (children, patients in hospice care, and those that need hospice care); cultural, spiritual, and ethical aspects of care; and palliative care delivery in the emergency department and in prehospital and international settings.

A practical understanding of palliative care in the emergency setting brings our desire to help one step closer for our sickest patients. Every practicing emergency clinician desires the same thing for their patient and their loved ones as we encounter their suffering: the best possible outcome in the context of an imperfect circumstance. We want to be a positive vehicle of help, support, and kindness to mitigate fear and instill hope. Hope that though we are not able to change the circumstance, we can optimize its outcome. We are trained to make that contribution in a skilled, empathic manner in the context of uncertainty, in unfamiliar surroundings with all under stress.

I thank all the authors of this book for their time and effort to bring palliative care to their colleagues and peers. They are among the truly committed. This book is dedicated to them and all of the emergency clinician palliative care mavericks that came before and will come ahead to build and evolve this incredible field of palliative care in the emergency setting.

Contributors

Kate Aberger, MD, FACEP
Medical Director
Division of Palliative Medicine and
Geriatrics
St. Joseph's Health
Paterson, NJ, USA

Daniel Bell, MD
Assistant Professor
Division of Palliative Medicine
Emory University School of
Medicine
Atlanta, GA, USA

Gretchen E. Bell, MD
Assistant Professor
Division of Palliative Medicine
Emory University School of
Medicine
Atlanta, GA, USA

Jason K. Bowman, MD
Instructor and Clinical Attending
Physician
Department of Emergency
Medicine
Department of Psychosocial
Oncology and Palliative Medicine
Brigham and Women's Hospital
Dana Farber Cancer Institute
Harvard Medical School
Boston, MA, USA

Laura Brachman, MD
Assistant Professor
Division of Palliative Medicine
Emory University School of
Medicine
Atlanta, GA, USA

Jay M. Brenner, MD
Associate Professor
Department of Emergency Medicine
SUNY-Upstate Medical University
Syracuse, NY, USA

Arthur Derse, MD, JD
Professor
Center for Bioethics and Medical
Humanities
Department of Emergency
Medicine
Medical College of Wisconsin
Milwaukee, WI, USA

**Paul L. DeSandre, DO,
FACEP, FAAHPM**
Associate Professor
Department of Emergency
Medicine
Department of Family and
Preventive Medicine,
Division of Palliative Medicine
Emory University School of
Medicine
Atlanta, GA, USA

Marie-Carmelle Elie, MD, FACEP, FCCM, RDMS
Professor & Chair
Department of Emergency Medicine
University of Alabama, Birmingham
Birmingham, AL, USA

Kirsten G. Engel, MD
Section of Palliative Care
Division of General Medicine
Beth Israel Deaconess Medical Center
Boston, MA, USA

Emilee Flynn, MD, MPH
Assistant Professor
Attending Physician, Pediatric Advanced Care Team
Children's Healthcare of Atlanta
Department of Pediatrics
Emory University School of Medicine
Atlanta, GA, USA

Alina M. Fomovska, MD
Assistant Professor
Department of Emergency Medicine
Jefferson University
Philadelphia, PA, USA

Rebecca Goett, MD, FACEP, FAAHPM
Associate Professor
Department of Emergency Medicine and Palliative Care
Rutgers New Jersey Medical School
Newark, NJ, USA

Eric Isaacs, MD
Professor
Department of Emergency Medicine
Zuckerberg San Francisco General Hospital
University of California, San Francisco
San Francisco, CA, USA

Lekshmi Kumar, MD, MPH
Associate Professor
Department of Emergency Medicine
Section of Prehospital and Disaster Medicine
Emory University School of Medicine
Atlanta, GA, USA

Joanne Kuntz, MD, FAAHPM, FACEP
Associate Professor
Department of Family and Preventive Medicine
Division of Palliative Medicine
Emory University School of Medicine
Atlanta, GA, USA

Sangeeta Lamba, MD, MS-HPEd
Professor
Department of Emergency Medicine
Rutgers New Jersey Medical School
Rutgers University
Newark, NJ, USA

Imad El Majzoub, MD
Consultant of Emergency Medicine
Associate Professor
Sheikh Shakhbout Medical City—
Mayo Clinic
Khalifa University
Abu Dhabi, United Arab Emirates

Julie Mitchell, DO
Assistant Professor
Department of Family and
Preventive Medicine
Division of Palliative Medicine
Emory University School of
Medicine
Atlanta, GA, USA

Clariliz Munet-Colón, MD
Department of Otolaryngology-HNS
University of Puerto Rico
San Juan, Puerto Rico

Carter Neugarten, MD
Assistant Professor
Departments of Internal Medicine
and Emergency Medicine, Section
of Palliative Care
Director of Palliative Emergency Care
Rush University Medical Center
Chicago, IL, USA

Kei Ouchi, MD, MPH
Assistant Professor
Department of Emergency
Medicine
Brigham and Women's Hospital
Harvard Medical School
Boston, MA, USA

Tammie E. Quest,MD, FAAHPM
Professor
Director, Emory Palliative
Care Center
Department of Family and
Preventive Medicine
Chief, Division of Palliative
Medicine
Department of Emergency
Medicine
Emory University School of
Medicine
Atlanta, GA, USA

Cynthia S. Romero, MD
Assistant Professor
Department of Emergency
Medicine
Section of Prehospital and Disaster
Medicine
Emory University School of
Medicine
Atlanta, GA, USA

Monique Schaulis, MD, MPH
Senior Physician
The Permanente Medical Group
Volunteer Clinical Faculty, UCSF
San Francisco, CA, USA

Ashley Shreves, MD
Department of Emergency
Medicine
Department of Palliative Care
Ochsner Medical Center
New Orleans, LA, USA

Danielle Stansky, MD
Resident Physician
Ronald O. Perelman Department
of Emergency Medicine
New York University School of
Medicine
New York, NY, USA

Audrey Tan, DO
Regional Medical Officer
Landmark Health
Optum Home and Community
New York, NY, USA

Liliana Viera-Ortiz, MD
Department of Surgery
University of Puerto Rico
San Juan, Puerto Rico

David Wang, MD
Director
Department of Palliative Medicine
Scripps Health
San Diego, CA, USA

Emily Zametkin, MBBS
Assistant
Department of Medicine
Palliative Care and Emergency
Medicine
University of Massachusetts Chan
Medical School—Baystate
Springfield, MA, USA

1 Here We Go Again

Jason K. Bowman

Case: A 72-year-old woman with advanced heart failure and oxygen-dependent chronic obstructive pulmonary disease presents to the emergency department (ED) with severe shortness of breath with blood pressure of 70/40 mmHg, heart rate of 140 beats per minute, respiratory rate of 40 per minute, and oxygen saturation of 85% on 2 L. On arrival to the ED, she is placed on noninvasive ventilation and administered furosemide 80 mg IV once. After 1 hour, she is clinically improved and able to be removed from the noninvasive ventilation. Radiographs and laboratory data are consistent with a new non-ST elevation myocardial infarction and heart failure exacerbation. She will be admitted to the intensive care unit. She reports that she lives alone in a senior living apartment, and that she has been having more trouble at home over the last month. The patient's neighbor was doing grocery shopping for her and getting her medications, but this individual was recently hospitalized as well. For the last 2 weeks she has been eating easy-to-reheat meals. She is widowed but has three adult children who live in the area. Over the last 6 months she has had three admissions to the hospital, and she does not have an advance care planning document.

What do you do now?

PRIMARY EMERGENCY DEPARTMENT PALLIATIVE CARE

Approximately 75% of all older patients visit an ED in the last 6 months of life, and over 50% will visit one in their final month of life. This case is representative of many patients seen in EDs: advanced age with multiple progressing chronic conditions that are life-limiting, limited social supports, and little if any advance care planning. Depending on community resources, outpatient providers (both primary care and specialists) may increasingly need to rely on EDs to evaluate these complex patients in the serious illness safety net. Unfortunately, many of these patients may suffer from poorly addressed physical, psychological, and social symptoms. Hospitalization can lead to invasive interventions that are frequently not aligned with their wishes. Expert, compassionate management of these challenging patients requires simultaneous disease-directed assessment and management, symptom management, and rapid but thoughtful exploration of goals of care in order to guide treatment decisions.

BACKGROUND

Palliative care focuses on optimizing quality of life throughout the illness spectrum by anticipating, preventing, and relieving suffering. Palliative care is interdisciplinary in nature, focused on the physical, spiritual, psychological, and social aspects of serious illness care—not only in medical management but also in navigating and leading challenging conversations with patients and families. Recognizing the value that palliative medicine offers, the American College of Emergency Physicians (ACEP) has recommended that providers "Don't delay in engaging available palliative and hospice services in the ED for patients likely to benefit."

PRIMARY PALLIATIVE CARE IN THE EMERGENCY DEPARTMENT

For various reasons, specialty-trained palliative medicine clinicians are not always available for ED consultation. Unfortunately, there already is a shortage of specialty-trained palliative providers for patients who might benefit, and this is expected to increase significantly in the coming decades.

One study estimated that by 2030 there will be one palliative medicine provider for every 26,000 patients in the United States. Globally, the WHO estimates that each year over 40,000,000 people around the world are in need of palliative care, yet only about 14% of them ever receive it. They believe the global need for palliative care will continue to grow. Given these statistics, there is increasing interest in and focus on training providers from many different specialties, including emergency medicine, in primary palliative care skills.

Providing primary palliative care in the ED requires a fundamental knowledge and set of practiced skills, in order to optimize serious illness care of ED patients. These span topics including interdisciplinary approaches to communication, symptom management, models of care, prognostication, ethical and legal issues, and other skills that should be learned and practiced by all medical providers (see Table 1.1). In 2018, a group of expert dual-trained ED-palliative clinicians and researchers expanded on this idea by describing a primary palliative medicine curriculum outline for ED training programs, based on the Accreditation Council for Graduate Medical Education (ACGME)'s "Milestones" framework.[1]

Primary palliative care skills are particularly vital in emergency medicine. Most patients arrive in the emergency department suffering from one or more symptoms, and many interactions with patients and/or their families will involve navigating challenging conversations. Yet historically,

TABLE 1.1 **Primary Palliative Care Skills**

Pain and Other Symptom Management	Care in the Final Hours of Life
Communication · Focused goals-of-care conversations · Breaking bad news · Death disclosure	Caregiver support Advance Care Planning
Family presence during resuscitation	Bereavement
Ethical and legal aspects of care	Caring for patients receiving hospice care
Withdrawing/withholding life-sustaining therapies	

emergency providers have received little or no training in these areas. Not surprisingly, surveyed ED clinicians express discomfort with caring for these challenging and vulnerable patients. Additionally, caring for patients with serious illness in the ED without the necessary full range of knowledge and skills can lead to provider distress and burnout, as well as avoidable patient suffering and care that are discordant with patient and family goals.

CASE DISCUSSION

The 72-year-old patient in the case study at the start of this chapter was effectively resuscitated in the ED and able to wean from noninvasive ventilation. Now she is awaiting an available intensive care bed. It is vitally important for clinicians caring for patients like her to pause and consider where the patient is along her global illness trajectory. She is elderly, has few supports, has two serious and potentially life-limiting medical conditions, and has been admitted numerous times in the past 6 months. She is facing a critical point not just in her hospital course but also in her life.

Recognizing this, then making a thoughtful and compassionate recommendation about best next steps for this patient will depend on the clinician's understanding of her values, hopes, and goals as they relate to her medical care, as well as appreciating the nature of her acute illness and being able to prognosticate her likely survival.

Both performing prognostication and effectively communicating it to patients and families can at baseline be quite challenging, and numerous aspects of emergency medicine care make it even harder. Providers in the ED do not have the benefit of longitudinal experience with patients or families, diagnostic uncertainty often is present at the time of the prognostication conversation, and predicting how a patient will respond to an acute potentially reversible event is challenging. Working in a high-distraction, multitasking environment as one prepares for and attempts to lead prognostication/goals-of-care conversations provides a continual challenge. Environmental factors such as crowdedness, noise, and lack of private spaces are also common issues in a busy ED. Despite the unique challenges to prognostication with ED patients, ED providers do have several potential tools to help them.

The first, entitled "The Surprise Question," was initially described by Murray in 2011 and involves providers asking themselves the question,

"Would I be surprised if this patient died in (e.g., hours, days, weeks, months) or during this hospitalization?" Subsequent studies have shown that answers to this question are predictive in numerous subsets of populations, including general patients in the ED[2] and heart failure patients in the ED specifically,[3] with negative predictive values of around 90%.

In patients with life-limiting, serious illness, a patient's ability to do everyday tasks is another valuable source of prognostic information. A number of validated functional performance scales used in the palliative care setting can assist clinicians in prognostication. When assessing performance status for the purposes of prognostication, the performance status should be assessed before and after symptom control. For example, pain or shortness of breath that is unmanaged may denote poor functional status in error. Oncologist Dr. David Karnofsky created a performance status scoring system in the 1960s for his oncology patients, and this later evolved into the modern "Palliative Performance Scale" created by Anderson et al. in 1996 and later updated in 2006.[4] This scale has been widely used, and subsequently validated in oncology, non-oncology, and heterogeneous populations for use in patients with life-limiting, advanced illness. The scale is depicted in Table 1.2 and is read from left to right starting with best ambulation and moving across to the right for each category. Knowing the patient's underlying primary illness (e.g., cancer, organ failure, dementia) and their performance status can help providers to estimate their progression along typical illness trajectory curves, such as the one depicted in Figure 1.1.[3]

Finally, though ED providers often have numerous things simultaneously vying for their time—and they are frequently interrupted—a brief review of any recent notes in the patient's chart from their specialist (e.g., oncologist, heart failure specialist, palliative care provider) can provide invaluable perspective on trajectory and prognosis. It can also help reveal if these providers have talked with the patient and/or their loved ones before about prognosis, goals, and so on. Similarly, a direct communication with the patient's specialist can provide valuable information and potentially prompt them to come to the ED to join the conversation with the patient and/or their loved ones. Even though the chart may report that specialist(s) have talked with the patient and/or their loved ones about prognosis, what the patient and family understood from the conversation at the time, let alone remember now in the ED, can vary greatly. Thus, it's critically

Illness trajectories	Emotional distress	Prognostic awareness
Ex. 1 Terminal cancer	High	Usually low
Ex. 2 Organ failure	Moderately ongoing	Variable
Ex. 3 Advanced dementia	Low	Usually high in surrogates

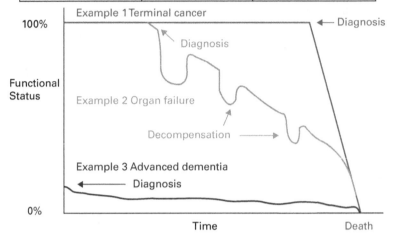

FIGURE 1.1. Illness trajectory, prognostic awareness and anticipated distress levels.

important to explore early in the patient's ED course their understanding of their prognosis.

In this case, even if the ED providers are unable to reach the patient's outpatient specialist providers, her known history and the ED evaluation already offer valuable information for prognostication. Given her comorbidities and her acute diagnoses, it would not be surprising if she did not survive this admission—and certainly not surprising if she didn't survive the next month or year. Additionally, even the brief information known about her challenges in managing alone at home put her Palliative Performance Score at 50%–60%. This, combined with the increasingly frequent rate of hospitalizations and her history of organ (heart) failure, also portends that she is far along in the typical heart failure illness trajectory. Collectively, these tools all suggest that the patient is likely nearing the end of her life.

Once a provider has an understanding of the patient's illness trajectory and prognosis, they can discuss this with the patient and explore their understanding of the illness (chronic and/or acute) and hopes, wishes, and

TABLE 1.2 The Palliative Performance Scale (PPS) Tool

PPS Level	Ambulation	Activity and Evidence of Disease	Self-Care	Intake	Conscious Level
100%	Full	Normal activity and work No evidence of disease	Full	Normal	Full
90%	Full	Normal activity and work Some evidence of disease	Full	Normal	Full
80%	Full	Normal activity with effort Some evidence of disease	Full	Normal or reduced	Full
70%	Reduced	Unable to do normal job/work Significant disease	Full	Normal or reduced	Full
60%	Reduced	Unable to do any work Extensive disease	Occasional assistance necessary	Normal or reduced	Full or confusion
50%	Mainly sit/lie	Unable to do most activity Extensive disease	Considerable assistance required	Normal or reduced	Full or confusion
40%	Mainly in bed	Unable to do any activity Extensive disease	Mainly assistance	Normal or reduced	Full or drowsy +/– Confusion
30%	Totally bed bound	Unable to do any activity Extensive disease	Total care	Minimal to sips	Full or drowsy +/– Confusion
20%	Totally bed bound	Unable to do any activity Extensive disease	Total care	Mouth care	Full or drowsy +/– Confusion
10%	Totally bed bound	Unable to do any activity Extensive disease	Total care		Drowsy or coma +/– Confusion
0%	Death	—	—	—	—

Source: Palliative Performance Scale (PPSv2) version 2. Victoria Hospice Society. https://victoriahospice.org/wp-content/uploads/2019/07/ppsv2_english_-_sample_-_dec_17.pdf

priorities given to it. There are numerous validated tools to help providers guide patients through these types of conversations. One commonly used example is the "REMAP" tool, first described by JW Childers et al. in 2017.[5] An example of how the tool could be used to guide a conversation with the specific patient in this case example scenario is described in Box 1.1.

BOX 1.1 **The REMAP Tool**

1. *Reframe.* "What is your understanding of what your doctors have told you about your health before today, and what explanations have you gotten here in the emergency department about what's causing your symptoms today?" If the patient's understanding appears to differ from the clinical realities, consider using a follow-up statement such as "Unfortunately, we're in a different place now, given the results of the tests we've done here in the emergency department today. Is it okay if we talk more about them and what we think is causing your symptoms?"

2. *Expect emotion.* Stop talking and listen! Consider responding to the patient's emotion directly. Examples of this include the following: "I can see you're really concerned about this. Is it okay if we talk a bit more about what this means for you?" or "I can't imagine what it's been like to hear all this news." Don't be afraid of silence. The patient's impression of her own health may be a lot different than what you're telling her now, and this may be a large emotional shock. After pausing, you could use a line such as "Tell me what's going through your mind."

3. *Map values.* Try to identify the patient's goals before making any recommendations. For example, you could ask her, "Given what we've just discussed about the challenging illnesses you're dealing with now, what's most important to you as we think about next steps?" More open-ended questions could also be helpful, such as simply, "What values and aspects of day-to-day life are most important to you?"

4. *Align with values.* "Now that I have a better understanding of what's important to you, let's talk a bit more about possible options for moving forward." If she shares a goal or wish that seems medically unfeasible, you can still align with their hope by saying something like "I wish that there was some way to make that possible . . ."

5. *Propose a plan.* It is often helpful to give specific recommendations, rather than simply a list of options. "From what you've told me about what's most important to you, I recommend . . . How does that sound to you?" Lead with the things you will do and explain how they fit into the patient's expressed values or wishes, rather than starting with what you will not do.

It is important to note that an important component of these conversations is making a recommendation. Interestingly, many providers report that they do not regularly make recommendations to patients and/or their loved ones. One possible reason for this is concern around appearing paternalistic or potentially compromising patient autonomy. However, research suggests that patients and families welcome compassionate guidance in the form of a recommendation informed by their expressed values, goals, and priorities. Additionally, not making a recommendation could bias the patient or their loved ones to choose interventions or care plans that providers believe are unlikely to help and will cause unnecessary suffering.[6]

Sometimes, even with the best guidance and support, patients and/or their loved ones are unable to make immediate decisions about their care. At the same time, the nature of the ED, and the potentially acute, unstable, or tenuous state of the patient, may not allow extended time for reflection and re-evaluation. A solution in some cases may be for the ED provider to offer to step out of the room and return in a few minutes. This allows the patient and family some precious time and space, and meanwhile the ED provider can check in on the other patients they're managing. Ultimately, if there is difficulty coming to a decision regarding goals of care, a palliative care specialist (if available) can provide excellent support to patient and provider alike. If a specialist is not available, or a consensus still cannot be reached, another option is a "time-limited trial," where an invasive and/ or potentially unhelpful intervention may be done temporarily to allow more time for trajectory clarification, reflection by the patient and family, and so on.

CASE CONCLUSION

For the patient in this case scenario vignette, the patient told the ED team that her primary goal was to remain home and avoid coming to the hospital again if possible. Although frail and increasingly unable to care for herself, she reported that she still enjoyed reading, seeing her local children and grandchildren, and calling friends on the telephone. She stated that she would not ever want to die hooked up to a ventilator or in a coma.

After exploring and understanding the patient's illness trajectory, prognosis, and goals and wishes, the ED team made an informed recommendation to admit her to the intensive care unit for medical optimization, a chance to confer a plan with outpatient heart failure physician and family, and plan for hospice evaluation with the goal of symptom control should the patient and family agree. Given the patient's wish to remain at home and avoid intubation, as well as her advanced disease and low likelihood of benefit from invasive resuscitation (such as in the event of cardiac arrest), the ED team also recommended a code status of "DNR/DNI" (do not resuscitate/do not intubate). She was admitted to the critical care unit for symptom management and monitoring, seen by her heart failure physician, and subsequently transferred to the floor. She was discharged home with hospice care after stabilization, additional conversations with the patient and her adult children, and ensuring that she had a safe home support system. The patient died peacefully at home, several weeks later.

In summary, primary palliative care skills are an essential part of expert emergency medicine practice. The environment of the ED presents numerous challenges in addition to those already inherent to trying to understand disease trajectory, prognosticate, and guide difficult conversations. However, successfully applying these skills can help avoid unnecessary physical and emotional suffering, and lead to more compassionate, holistic, and patient-aligned emergency medicine care.

"The task of medicine is to cure sometimes, treat often, and comfort always."
Ambroise Pare, 16th-century French surgeon

KEY POINTS

- Assess the patient's disease trajectory and use data, including performance status, to prognosticate.
- Seek to understand the patient's values, hopes, and goals.
- Use your expert opinion from evaluating seriously ill patients to make a recommendation.
- Recognize that not all problems can be solved in the ED, including understanding and aligning prognosis with patient and family goals. In these cases, consider a time-limited trial of more intensive interventions, as indicated.

- Consider using a validated tools and communication paradigm in palliative care to help you guide the patient (and/or family) through these conversations.

Further Reading

1. Shoenberger J, Lamba S, Goett R, et al. Development of hospice and palliative medicine knowledge and skills for emergency medicine residents: Using the Accreditation Council for Graduate Medical Education milestone framework. *AEM Education and Training.* 2018;2(2):130–145. doi:10.1002/aet2.10088.

2. Ouchi K, Jambaulikar G, George N, et al. The "surprise question" asked of emergency physicians may predict 12-month mortality among older emergency department patients. *Journal of Palliative Medicine.* 2018;21(2):236–240. doi:10.1089/jpm.2017.0192.

3. Aaronson E, George N, Ouchi K, et al. The surprise question can be used to identify heart failure patients in the emergency department who would benefit from palliative care. *Journal of Pain and Symptom Management.* 2019;57(5):944–951. doi:10.1016/j.jpainsymman.2019.02.007.

4. Anderson F, Downing G, Hill J, et al. Palliative performance scale (PPS): A new tool. *Journal of Palliative Care.* 1996;12(1):5–11. doi:10.1177/082585979601200102.

5. Childers JW, Back AL, Tulsky JA, et al. REMAP: A framework for goals of care conversations. *Journal of Oncology Practice.* 2017;13(10): e844–850. doi:10.1200/JOP.2016.018796.

6. Jacobsen J, Blinderman C, Alexander Cole C, Jackson V. "I'd recommend . . .": How to incorporate your recommendation into shared decision making for patients with serious illness. *Journal of Pain and Symptom Management.* 2018;55(4):1224–1230. doi:10.1016/j.jpainsymman.2017.12.488.

7. Wang D. Beyond code status: Palliative care begins in the emergency department. *Annals of Emergency Medicine.* 2017;69(4):437–443. doi:10.1016/j.annemergmed.2016.10.027.

8. Palliative Care and End-of-Life Care—A Consensus Report. National Quality Forum. Published April 2012. Accessed November 2019. https://www.qualityforum.org/Publications/2012/04/Palliative_Care_and_End-of-Life_Care—A_Consensus_Report.aspx

9. Palliative Care—Key Facts. World Health Organization. Published August 2020. https://www.who.int/news-room/fact-sheets/detail/palliative-care

10. Connor, Stephen. Global Atlas of Palliative Care 2nd Edition Global Atlas of Palliative Care at the End of Life Global Atlas of Palliative Care 2nd Edition; 2020.

11. Quill TE, Abernethy AP. Generalist plus specialist palliative care—Creating a more sustainable model. *New England Journal of Medicine.* 2013;368:1173–1175. doi:10.1056/NEJMp1215620.

12. Kamal AH, Bull JH, Swetz KM, et al. Future of the palliative care workforce: Preview to an impending crisis. *The American Journal of Medicine.* 2016;130(2):113–114. doi:10.1016/j.amjmed.2016.08.046.

13. Murray S, Boyd K. Using the "surprise question" can identify people with advanced heart failure and COPD who would benefit from a palliative care approach. *Palliative Medicine.* 2011;25(4):382. doi:10.1177/0269216311401949.

14. Ouchi K, George N, Schuur J, et al. Goals-of-care conversations for older adults with serious illness in the emergency department: Challenges and opportunities. *Annals of Emergency Medicine.* 2019;74(2):276–284. doi:10.1016/j.annemergmed.2019.01.003.

15. Paske JRT, DeWitt S, Hicks R, Semmens S, Vaughan L. Palliative care and rapid emergency screening tool and the Palliative Performance Scale to predict survival of older adults admitted to the hospital from the emergency department. *American Journal of Hospice Palliative Care.* 2021 Jul;38(7):800–806.

2 Time Waits for No One

Emily Zametkin and Kei Ouchi

Case: A 78-year-old man with advanced Parkinson's disease, congestive heart failure, hypertension, multiple cerebral vascular events, and a recent hip fracture status post internal fixation presents to the emergency department (ED) with fever and cough. He is bedbound and is unable to communicate his needs at baseline. He has a gastrostomy tube for artificial nutrition and medications. He has had four admissions in the last 6 months. His wife is at the bedside and feels that he is suffering. She says that he is getting progressively worse, and she asks you how long you think he has to live.

What do you do now?

TRAJECTORIES AND PROGNOSTICATION

Presentation to the ED often represents an inflection point in the advanced illness trajectory and offers an opportunity to address "big picture" questions about goals of care, quality of life, and priorities moving forward. To make an informed decision, the patient and family must be able to answer the question: *"What have you heard from your care team about where you are with your illness?"* Being able to understand the patient's "big picture" can be thought of as a trajectory. Exploring the common trajectories of serious illnesses typically encountered in the ED can be useful for prognosticating. How much time one has left on their "big picture" trajectory can be thought of as the prognosis. Units of time such as minutes, hours, days, weeks, or years can help patients, families, and other clinicians make decisions about what is next. Lunney and Lynn identified four common disease trajectories to describe the four common "big pictures" that patients experience: (1) sudden illness, (2) terminal illness, (3) organ failure, and (4) debility. The trajectories are based on studies of Medicare beneficiaries and serve as a useful starting point.

On a *sudden illness trajectory*, the patient is at or near 100% functional status, and a sudden, devastating acute event occurs. Examples include cardiac arrest, trauma, or stroke. The patient experience is one of acute and precipitous decline with uncertain potential for recovery. Families are often asked to make difficult decisions quickly, without time to process shock or grief. The type of sudden event, as well as the patient's health status before the event, greatly impacts prognosis. After cardiac arrest, typical survival to discharge after emergency medical service–treated, out-of-hospital cardiac arrest is roughly 10% for all adults, while survival is just over 20% for in-hospital cardiac arrest. For an ED presentation such as trauma, the long-term consequences of traumatic injuries vary widely based on the health and functional status of a patient pre-injury. Studies have shown that pre-injury functional status has more to do with survival and disability than the actual injuries sustained. Patients with low functional status tend to have higher rates of in-hospital mortality, are more likely to be discharged to a rehabilitation or nursing facility, and are twice as likely to have poor functional outcomes.

On a *terminal illness trajectory*, also known as an advanced cancer trajectory, the patient has less than 100% of function but is living with advanced cancer and is often receiving cancer-directed therapies. At some point along that trajectory, the patient begins to have a moderately abrupt functional decline that continues over weeks to months and is not significantly modified by cancer-directed therapy, with progressive weakness until death. Patients who have lived with advanced cancer for months or years may expect that treatments will continue to prolong their life and may be hoping that new treatments will become available. Unlike other disease states, which are characterized by exacerbations and some recovery, incurable cancer usually involves a period of relative stability followed by a rapid, brief, and dramatic decline. In a study of patients with metastatic or local cancer who presented to the ED, over half were admitted to the hospital, and the one-year overall survival of patients following presentation was 7.3 months. Over 20% of these patients died within the first month. Presentations for shortness of breath were associated with a poorer prognosis.

On an *organ failure trajectory*, patients have some vital solid organ impairment such as heart, liver, kidney, or lung failure. On this trajectory, without transplantation, patients will experience periods of sharp decline and recovery with exacerbations of congestive heart failure, end-stage renal disease, end-stage liver failure, or chronic obstructive pulmonary disease. Patients have recurrent episodes of an abrupt decline and recovery with the use of medications or devices. The expectation on this trajectory by patients and families is often that they will be "saved" this time, just like previous times. Unfortunately, each exacerbation ends in a worsening function, leading to a gradual decline that may be hard for patients and families to recognize. It is uniquely challenging to predict which hospitalization will end with a person's death or result in a quality of life that is not acceptable to the patient.

Progressive heart failure, for example, is marked by a slow decline punctuated by acute exacerbations and temporary recovery to states, usually at a lower functional level. Increased rates of hospitalization, progressive increases in diuretics, reduced function, and the initiation of ionotropic therapy are indicators of decline. Mortality in the year following an ED visit for an exacerbation of symptoms is associated with increasing age, likely due to the duration of illness and overall health status. Like chronic heart failure, patients with chronic obstructive pulmonary disease tend to experience acute periods of decompensation followed by partial recovery and relative stability. Lack of further treatment options, functional decline, frequency of exacerbations, hospitalizations, and increasing oxygen requirements are indicators of poor prognosis. In patients with chronic kidney disease, albumin level, age, concomitant peripheral vascular disease, and dementia are associated with expedited mortality.

It can be useful to share the expected organ failure trajectory with patients and their families so that they can appreciate the overall decline that is anticipated with these chronic, terminal illnesses. Asking how functional status has changed in the previous months, especially after discharge from a hospital or rehabilitation center, can help patients and families reflect on how things have changed. This can also be used to open a discussion about goals and expectations.

On a *debility trajectory*, patients experience a steady and gradual decline that may be particularly challenging for caregivers. Months and often years of deterioration occur, punctuated by acute illness and recovery. Patients with dementia often follow this pattern of decline. It can be difficult to identify if patients are living in a way that they would find acceptable and to recognize that subtle changes may signal that death is imminent. Patients with severe dementia (FAST stage 7) are often profoundly disabled and at high risk of death, yet very few are referred to hospice in the last 6 months of their lives because of the difficulty of predicting survival. The median survival time after a diagnosis of Alzheimer's disease ranges from 3 to 12 years, and many patients are fully dependent for the majority of their remaining time. For patients admitted to nursing homes, the median survival is 1.3 years. Common complications include lack of nutrition, aspiration episodes, and infections such as pneumonia and urinary tract infections. An increase in the frequency of presentations to the ED often signals a more rapid decline.

True emergencies, such as sepsis or respiratory failure, which present in patients on any trajectory, require immediate decisions to be made that will ultimately determine the prognosis for the patient. These unexpected events carry significant mortality and morbidity. Mortality in patients admitted to the hospital with sepsis varies widely across studies. The very definition of sepsis changes depending on inclusion and exclusion criteria. In one study looking at all medical and surgical admissions of septic adults to three urban academic centers in an American city, 14.8% died during

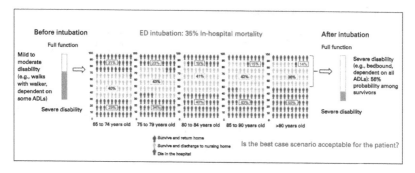

FIGURE 2.1. Outlook after emergency department intubation in seriously ill older adults.

Ouchi K, Lawton AJ, Bowman J, Bernacki R, George N. Managing Code Status Conversations for Seriously Ill Older Adults in Respiratory Failure. *Ann Emerg Med.* 2020 12; 76(6):751–756. PMID: 32747084. https://www.annemergmed.com/article/S0196-0644(20)30410-8/pdf

Reprinted with permission.

hospitalization. According to the same study, there has been a marked decrease in deaths from 2010 to 2015; however, in the population of survivors, readmission rates to the hospital were high. Emergent intubation in older adults, in particular, is often associated with poor prognosis. In one study, 35% of older adults intubated in the ED died during hospitalization, with mortality increasing markedly with age, reaching 50% among those aged 90 years (Figure 2.1). For those who died in the hospital, the median time to death is 3 days. Sepsis and myocardial infarction in those intubated were more highly associated with mortality. When older adults are intubated and survive the hospitalization, the functional decline is expected. The majority of older adults intubated died within a year, and over 70% were discharged to a skilled nursing facility, long-term acute care hospital, or hospice. Emergency medicine (EM) providers must forecast not only the expected mortality but also the functional prognosis when discussing the overall prognosis of the patients in the ED.

In the context of the four trajectories, seriously ill adults often present in two ways: acute decompensation or a subtle change in health status that signals a more rapid decline may be ahead. During an acute decompensation, EM providers frequently face questions about prognosis and trajectory for seriously ill patients visiting the ED (Figure 2.2). During this acute decompensation, "crisis communication" is used to rapidly make

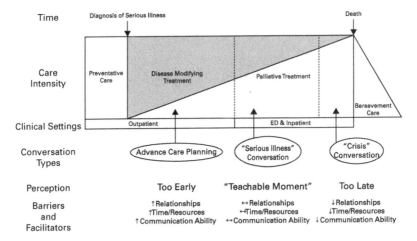

FIGURE 2.2. Types of goals-of-care conversations in the emergency department.

Ouchi K, George N, Schuur JD, Aaronson EL, Lindvall C, Bernstein E, Sudore RL, Schonberg MA, Block SD, Tulsky JA. Goals-of-Care Conversations for Older Adults With Serious Illness in the Emergency Department: Challenges and Opportunities. *Ann Emerg Med.* 2019; 74(2):276–284. PMID: 30770207. https://www.ncbi.nlm.nih.gov/pmc/articles/PMC6714052/. Reprinted with permission.

important decisions that will ultimately determine the course of treatment. During less dramatic presentations (e.g., 30-day readmission for refractory symptoms related to heart failure), "serious illness conversations" are used to reformulate goals in the context of a new reality of illness. Both types of conversations rely on accurate bedside assessment, the rapid establishment of rapport with patients and families, and the ability of a provider to comfortably convey difficult news. Patients, families, or other clinicians may ask, "How long do you think they have to live?" as they weigh their options. Estimates about the overall health of a patient are vital in determining what interventions should be offered in the acute setting and can be used to set expectations with patients and families. Despite a provider's potential fear about discussing the end of life, patients and families often expect to have conversations about the anticipated decline and life expectancy and rely on the information gained to prepare for impending disability and death. EM providers are experts at determining "sick" from "not sick" and are adept at making immediate, comprehensive assessments of a patient, often with a lack of information.

In the case presented above, a patient on the debility trajectory has presented with signs and symptoms of an infection. This patient has had a precipitous decline: recurrent hospitalizations, a recent hip fracture, and a significant infection. These changes signal alteration in the trajectory and prognosis for this patient. Time is now short. Relaying this information to the wife in the ED would enable her to make critical decisions about treatment and disposition.

PROGNOSTICATION TOOLS

Evidence-based tools exist to aid in prognostication, specific to certain patient populations and medical conditions, yet many are too cumbersome to use in the ED. A few of these tools, however, can be useful because of their practicality and simplicity. The Palliative Performance Scale (PPS) is a simple assessment of function, activity, intake, and level of consciousness that can be used to predict survival and rate of meaningful decline in patients with a terminal illness. Unlike other predictive tools, the PPS is not reliant on laboratory testing or physician estimates for survival, making it a simple adjuvant to bedside clinical assessment. It can be used as a "reality check" for patients and EM providers, especially during disposition planning.

The "surprise question" is a simple screening tool used to identify patients who may benefit from a goals-of-care conversation and a palliative approach to care. Providers ask themselves, "Would I be surprised if this patient were to die in the next 6–12 months?" If the answer is "no," then this should trigger a conversation about patient priorities early during assessment and treatment. In a systematic review and meta-analysis of the use of the surprise question at identifying patients at the end of life, there was a wide range of sensitivity and specificity for survival. Clinicians were better at predicting which patients would survive compared to choosing those who would die. Interestingly, clinicians were no better at predicting imminent death compared to death over a 6-month or 12-month period. In a study looking at the accuracy of predictions for death in the next 1 month made by EM providers admitting patients ≥65 years old to the hospital, the question had a sensitivity of 43% and a specificity of 82%. The tool, therefore, is not sensitive enough to be used in isolation, but it is easily integrated into practice and can empower EM providers to identify patients who will be unlikely to benefit from certain interventions while in the hospital. Further, allowing EM providers to verbalize their overall clinical impression may empower them to act on their worries.

Additional prognostic tools include the Palliative Prognostic Score, the Prognosis in Palliative Care Study Scores, and the Palliative Performance Index, but these have been validated for specific diseases and require data that may not be readily available in the ED. EM providers should be aware that these tools exist and have a general understanding of what characteristics are associated with limited survival, such as symptoms limiting daily activities. Acute care physicians cannot and should not be reliant on complex, disease-specific models for predicting survival. General gestalt about the overall health of a patient, coupled with a thorough physical exam, should guide decisions made about interventions that may affect prognosis. To facilitate shared decision-making, providers must feel comfortable making assessments at the bedside and communicating openly about whether treatments will enable patients to live in a way that would be acceptable to them.

COMMUNICATION IN THE EMERGENCY DEPARTMENT

EM providers are in a unique position to share prognostic information because patients must confront the complexities of living with serious illness at a time when daily life is abruptly interrupted. Patients and families may be most receptive to "big picture" conversations during crisis encounters. Sharing prognostic information with patients is not only expected but is critical during communication in the context of serious illness, especially when healthcare decisions must be made imminently.

Prognostication, conflict mediation, empathic communication, and family-centered aspects of care have been identified as core competencies for providers who deal with critically ill patients. Patients should be asked what they know about their prognosis and how much information they would like to receive in regard to survival. It is recommended that patients be allowed to express how and to what extent family members should be involved in decision-making. Best practices for sharing prognostic information include acknowledging uncertainty when predicting survival and decline as well as making explicit that prognosis is fluid and may change from hour to hour. Information should be delivered at an appropriate pace, with room for adjustments along the way. EM providers should anticipate and prepare for dealing with difficult emotions, with an understanding that fear and anxiety can limit how much information can be processed over the course of one conversation. These interactions are admittedly challenging, but the Serious Illness Conversation Guide, EM Talk, and other resources provide roadmaps for providers (Table 2.1).

PROGNOSTICATION CHALLENGES

Every ED visit is an opportunity to discuss prognosis, yet barriers exist that make these conversations difficult. Challenges to effective prognostication in the ED include lack of provider training, difficulty assessing patients with multiple serious medical problems that compound one another, and insecurity around interpreting and delivering survival data in a way that is relatable to patients. Prognostication is emotionally difficult and time intensive.

EM providers often wrestle with how to start these conversations and may find it easier to assume other members of the care team are responsible for these discussions. Yet it is critical that every EM provider take ownership of the process of educating patients and empowering them to make medical decisions in line with their goals. Barriers to open conversations include fears of making patients upset, causing loss of hope, trepidation over perceived trespassing into other specialties' territories, and a lack of resources available to address needs that are identified. There is also a wide spectrum of opinion, much of which is dictated by culture and personal experience of loss, which determines the willingness of clinicians to estimate how and over what period of time death will occur.

In our time-pressured practice environment, the default is to provide life-sustaining treatment, regardless of the likelihood of acceptable outcomes for patients. When time is limited and a patient's history is unknown, the assumption is to do everything and defer to inpatient teams to determine goals in the context of a new grim reality. Even when conversations result in the decision to withdraw invasive ventilation or transition to inpatient hospice, there are numerous challenges to implementing these plans in many EDs.

TABLE 2.1   **Emergency Department Code Status Conversation Guide**

Goal: Make patient-centered recommendations regarding incubation for patients who may be at high risk for poor outcomes. After establishing that <u>advance directive does not exist</u>, complete the following steps:

Steps	What to Say
Elicit understanding	I wish we met under different circumstances. Your [father] is very sick and we have to decide quickly about [his] care. What have you heard about what happened today?
Break bad news	**Ask permission:** I am afraid I have serious news. Would it be OK if I share? **Disclose:** Your [father] is having a very difficult time breathing due to a [severe pneumonia]. With his serious health issues, I am worried that things may not go well, and it's possible [he] could even die.
Align	We need to **work together quickly** to make the best decisions for [his] care.
Baseline function	To decide which treatments might help [his] the most, I need to know more about [him]: What **type of activities** was [he] doing day to day before this illness?
Values *Use question(s) as appropriate*	Has [he] **expressed wishes** about the type of medical care [he] would or wouldn't want? How might [he] **feel if treatments today led to: Inability** to return to [his] favorite activities? Inability to care for [himself] as much as [he] does? What **abilities are so crucial** that [he] wouldn't consider life worth living if [he] lost them? **How much** would [he] be willing to go through for the possibility of more time? Are there states [he] would consider **worse than dying?**
Summarize	What I heard is that your [father] considered_____ most important, and that [he] would consider treatments that result in _____ unacceptable. **Did I get that right?**

TABLE 2.1 **Continued**

	Based on what you've shared with me, **we would recommend:** · Intensive treatment focused on comfort; <u>or</u> · Intensive treatment focus on recovering from illness
	We **will use** all available medical treatments that we think will help [his] recover from this illness. For [him], this means:
Recommendation	· Supporting [his] body in recovering from this illness without treatments that could make [him] more uncomfortable, while do everything we can to assure that [he] is comfortable and peaceful; <u>or</u> · Supporting [his] body in recovering from this illness with intensive treatments, including ventilators, while also doing everything we can to assure that [he] is as comfortable as possible. I worry that even with maximum care, [his] body may still tire out. The admitting teams will support you over the coming days with upcoming decisions.
	Does this sound ok?
	Document the conversation

Source: Ouchi K, Lawton AJ, Bowman J, Bernacki R, George N. Managing Code Status Conversations for Seriously Ill Older Adults in Respiratory Failure. *Ann Emerg Med*. 2020 12; 76(6):751–756. PMID: 32747084. https://www.annemergmed.com/article/S0196-0644(20)30410-8/pdf
Reprinted with permission.

Despite these palpable barriers, both unique to emergency medicine and universal across disciplines, patients expect and are entitled to open, honest conversations about likely outcomes. Serious consequences of avoiding these conversations include providing care not consistent with goals, increasing healthcare costs without benefit, decreasing quality of life, prolonging death and suffering, and negatively impacting bereavement for families. Sharing prognostic information in the ED enables patients to begin to think about their goals of care at a critical juncture in their illness trajectories.

CONCLUSION

Prognosticating in the ED is a critical aspect of decision-making. In providing the best care for our patients, we should anticipate deterioration, offer interventions that will lead to acceptable outcomes for patients and families, and address psychosocial needs in the ED. This is often challenging, given patient volume, lack of control over environmental factors, and the possibility of a rapidly changing clinical picture. Nevertheless, prognostication is a skill that can be developed, and there are tools readily available to aid in decision-making and communication. Patients do not expect certainty but do desire transparency. EM providers are in a unique position to shape the course of hospitalization in the context of patient preferences and prognosis. Using the tools described above, we can empower patients to make medical decisions most consistent with their values.

> **KEY POINTS**
>
> · Prognosticating is a critical component of decision-making in the ED.
> · Diseases have specific, predictable trajectories.
> · Tools exist to aid in prognosticating for patients with serious illness.
> · Communicating prognosis is a necessary skill that can be learned.

Further Reading
1. Bernacki RE, Block SD. Communication about serious illness care goals: A review and synthesis of best practices. *JAMA Intern Med.* 2014;174(12):1994. doi:10.1001/jamainternmed.2014.5271.
2. Glare PA, Sinclair CT. Palliative medicine review: Prognostication. *J Palliat Med.* 2008;11(1):84–103. doi:10.1089/jpm.2008.9992.
3. Grudzen CR, Emlet LL, Kuntz J, Shreves A, Zimny E, Gang M, Schaulis M, Schmidt S, Isaacs E, Arnold R. EM talk: Communication skills training for emergency medicine patients with serious illness. *BMJ Support Palliat Care.* 2016;6(2):219–224. doi:10.1136/bmjspcare-2015-000993.
4. Hancock K, Clayton JM, Parker SM, Wal der S, Butow PN, Carrick S, Currow D, Ghersi D, Glare P, Hagerty R, Tattersall MH. Truth-telling in discussing

prognosis in advanced life-limiting illnesses: A systematic review. *Palliat Med.* 2007;21(6):507–517. doi:10.1177/0269216307080823.

5. Lakin JR, Jacobsen J. Softening our approach to discussing prognosis. *JAMA Intern Med.* 2019;179(1):5. doi:10.1001/jamainternmed.2018.5786.

6. Lunney JR, Lynn J, Hogan C. Profiles of older Medicare decedents. *J Am Geriatr Soc.* 2002;50(6):1008–1012. doi:10.1046/j.1532-5415.2002.50268.

7. Ouchi K, George N, Schuur JD, Aaronson EL, Lindvall C, Bernstein E, Sudore RL, Schonberg MA, Block SD, Tulsky JA. Goals-of-care conversations for older adults with serious illness in the emergency department: Challenges and opportunities. *Annals of Emergency Medicine.* 2019;74(2):276–284. doi:10.1016/j.annemergmed.2019.01.003.

8. Smith AK, McCarthy E, Weber E, Cenzer IS, Boscardin J, Fisher J, Covinsky K. Half of older Americans seen in emergency department in last month of life; most admitted to the hospital, and many die there. *Health Affairs.* 2012;31(6):1277–1285.

3 We Are in a Different Place

Julie Mitchell and Joanne Kuntz

Case: A 46-year-old male with amyotrophic lateral sclerosis (ALS) presents to the emergency department (ED) with progressive shortness of breath. He is currently using a home noninvasive ventilator 22 hours per day, which has been increasing over the last month when he only needed it during the nighttime for 12 hours. He now states that he needs it almost continuously. In the ED, he is able to be off of noninvasive ventilation for no more than 10–15 minutes without reporting severe shortness of breath but is able to communicate clearly. In the ED, he has a blood gas measurement of pH 7.31; PCO_2 60; bicarbonate 23. His mother is at the bedside and reports that he seems very lethargic at home when he is not on the noninvasive ventilator. Due to long periods of use of the noninvasive home ventilator, his mother reports that his eating has diminished as well over the last month and she believes he is losing weight.

What do you do now?

GOALS-OF-CARE DISCUSSIONS

ALS is a progressive, terminal neurodegenerative disease characterized by loss of upper and lower motor neurons, resulting in a loss of physical, respiratory, speech, and swallowing functions. The onset of ALS involves muscle weakness or stiffness as early symptoms. Continued weakness, wasting, and paralysis of the limbs and trunk, as well as muscles that control vital functions such as speech, swallowing, and breathing, are evidence of progression. Most patients die from respiratory failure approximately 2 to 5 years after the onset of symptoms.

The American Academy of Neurology has developed ALS quality measures to address gaps in patient care and to overcome the underuse of evidence-based therapies for patients with ALS. They help to identify treatments that improve both longevity and quality of life; for example, enhanced survival and increased quality of life have been documented with use of noninvasive ventilation. For those who wish to pursue tracheostomy and invasive ventilation, quality of life may be preserved, though potentially with higher burden to caregivers. Enteral feeding also likely prolongs survival. These guidelines also encourage referral to multidisciplinary ALS clinics with a goal to plan for complex care needs using a patient-centered approach to proactive decision-making; this is achieved with a thorough goals-of-care discussion. The ideal time for these discussions to occur is in a calm setting prior to an acute decline or exacerbation—in this case, during a routine multidisciplinary clinic visit—so that decisions can be made prior to any crises that may require more urgent decision-making. Unfortunately, for a variety of factors this may not occur, and the patient presents to the ED with an acute decline or exacerbation where critical decisions must be made. Thus, the ED is a common setting for these life-altering dialogues to take place. Similar to other important procedural skills, a goals-of-care conversation is a critical skill that has specific steps that are key to a high-quality result. When we approach a goals-of-care conversation as a procedural skill and break it down into steps, we can become more fluid with practice and continued emphasis on the individual steps. As with any new procedural skill, the first step is preparation and ensuring all the necessary pieces are in place.

Preparation is an important step prior to any high-stakes conversation. Keys steps in preparation include gathering all the necessary information, including the right people for the discussion and providing an environment that will provide privacy and comfort for those involved. Gathering the necessary information includes a review of the patient's medical history and awareness of any available prognostic information. Ideally, a discussion with the ED provider, consultants, and primary physician or other involved specialists can provide a consistent message to the patient. Reviewing advance care planning documentation if available is also critical, as this can help guide your discussion, especially if the patient is not in a state to participate. This document may also identify the patient's appointed healthcare agent, who is the patient's legal surrogate decision maker in the event he or she is unable to contribute.

Environmental challenges to have goals-of-care conversations in the ED are many. While these discussions are best held in a quiet, comfortable environment that provides everyone—patient, family, clinicians—an opportunity to sit down, the ED rarely allows for this. If the patient is in a hallway area, the clinician should try, if even only temporarily, to move the patient to a more private setting. If the patient is in a shared room, the curtain should be pulled, and the clinicians should speak loud enough for the patient and family to hear but not others. Invite all participants in the meeting to introduce themselves and their relationship to the patient. Confirm that the necessary people are present. In the ED this may mean waiting until an important family member can arrive or including them via phone or video conference. It is important to note that those present or most available may not be the legal healthcare surrogate as outlined by state law if the patient is unable to participate or has not previously completed an advance directive.

Assess understanding of illness. No assumptions should be made throughout a goals-of-care discussion. Determine what the patient and family already know. "What have you heard from your care team about where you are with your illness?" Sometimes the patient or family is well informed, and they have a good understanding and prognostic awareness. They provide their own reframe in that sense. Other times you need to deliver serious news. Asking permission to share what you know is an important next step. "Would it be ok if I share with you what I understand?" This allows them some control back and helps you know if they are ready to hear the new information. Regardless of what the medical record states with regard to prior conversations as documented by other members of the healthcare team, what they have been *told* is not necessarily what they have *heard*.

Deliver medical information to facilitate shared decision-making. It is important to present medical information as clearly and succinctly as possible. Speak slowly and deliberately, avoiding medical jargon. Present the big picture and avoid getting caught up in the details of medicine that will likely be lost on the layperson. Use of the word "dying" is one that is often avoided, though powerful in helping the layperson realize the gravity of the situation if appropriate.

Delivering prognosis is challenging but important. Often, the most critical piece of information to help patients and families is your prognostic estimation. Prognosis often falls into one of three categories: uncertain, time based, or function based. The Serious Illness Conversation Guide has three useful prognostic statements that are generalizable to almost all clinical situations involving serious illness:

- *Uncertain*: "It can be difficult to predict what will happen with your illness. I hope you will continue to live well for a long time, but I'm worried that you could get sick quickly, and I think it is important to prepare for that possibility."
- *Time*: "I wish we were not in this situation, but I am worried that time may be as short as ___ (express a range, such as days to weeks, weeks to months, months to a year)."
- *Function*: "I hope that this is not the case, but I'm worried that this may be as strong as you will feel, and things are likely to get more difficult."

REMAP is a talking map or guide that provides a framework for a goals-of-care discussion. (See Table 3.1.)

1. *Reframe why the status quo isn't working.* You may need to discuss serious news (e.g., a scan result) first. "Given this news, it seems like a good time to talk about what to do now." "We're in a different place."
2. *Expect emotion and empathize.* Expect emotion and allow for silence; this gives the patient and family time to experience the emotion. Often, people will fill the silence with their thoughts or

TABLE 3.1 **REMAP: Goals of Care, Late in the Illness**

STEP	WHAT YOU SAY OR DO
REFRAME Why the status quo isn't working.	*"There is something I'd like to put on our agenda today."* *"We're in a different place."* *"This is a point where some treatments could do more harm than good."* You may have needed to give serious news first; that's a separate task.
EXPECT EMOTION respond with empathy.	*"It sounds like you are worried about [your family]." [Name the patient's emotion]* *"I can see how much you love your [son]."* *"You have worked so hard to do the right thing."*
MAP OUT big picture values, what's important.	*"Can we step back, think about what you are hoping for, and try to find a good option for you?"* *"Given this situation, what's most important for you now?"* *"Have you ever thought about what if things don't go the way you want?"*
ALIGN yourself & team with the patient's values.	*"It sounds like the most important issues to you are [spending time with your family, being comfortable, and enjoying your garden]"* *"By planning ahead, we can avoid some things you said you didn't want."* Reflect the patient's values.
PLAN medical treatments that match the patient's values.	*"Thank you for talking to me about this. I will talk to your team and come back later today with a plan."* *"For this situation, here are some things that I can do now . . . "*

ask questions that will easily bridge you to the natural next steps in conversation. Prior to continuing discussion, acknowledge and validate reactions and emotions. Frequent emotions encountered include acceptance, uncertainty, and anger. Using empathic statements to respond to these can help to normalize the process. "This must be very hard. I can't imagine how hard this must be for you."

3. *Map out what is important.* As stated earlier, the intent of a goals-of-care discussion is to ensure that the care provided aligns with patient values. Learning what is most important to them in the context of an accurate understanding of their illness trajectory not only clarifies patient priorities but also demonstrates the provider's interest in learning more about the patient as an individual. Once again, ask for permission to move forward. "Can we talk about what this means?"; "Given this situation, what's most important?"; "As you think about the future, what concerns you or worries you?" As you hear the answers to these questions, you will be able to identify the patient's values. Make mental note of what you hear. If you hear something like "I don't want to be a burden," explore further, asking "Tell me more." In the case described here, the patient is able to communicate and we can hear directly from him. In situations when the patient cannot participate, the provider should explore if the surrogate has had prior discussions about the "what ifs" with the patient. This patient, for example, may have had advance care planning discussions if he were a patient in a multidisciplinary ALS clinic, laying the groundwork for your current encounter. Additionally, it is important to frame questions to the surrogate to encourage them to respond from the perspective of the patient. "What would your son think if he could hear what we are saying?" Acknowledge the emotion associated with this, such as how difficult this must be for a mother to have to bear.

4. *Align with patient values.* This is where the provider summarizes the various priorities that they have identified. Again, demonstrating that they have been hearing and acknowledging what matters most now. Reflect to the patient and family what has been heard. Examples might be: "As I listen, it sounds like what's important

is . . . "; "I think we can help you not experience pain, spend more time with . . . " If the patient or family remark on things they don't want or don't want to do you might respond by saying "by planning ahead, we can avoid things like . . ."

5. *Plan treatments to match values.* This is the time at which the provider suggests a plan moving forward based on the values described. Once again, asking for permission, "May I make a recommendation?"; "Here are things we can do now . . ."; "For this situation, here are some things that would help. What do you think?" Once you have made all the recommendations of what *should be done based on values heard,* it may be appropriate to summarize treatments or procedures you are not recommending. Mutually decide with the patient on the steps necessary to achieve the stated goals. Common issues that may be discussed include future hospitalizations or intensive care unit (ICU) stays, diagnostic tests, do-not-resuscitate status, medically administered hydration and nutrition, antibiotics or blood products, and home support (home hospice) or placement. When trying to decide among various treatment options, a good rule of thumb is that if the intervention in question will not help toward meeting the stated goals, then it should be discontinued, not offered, or not initiated.

CASE CONCLUSION

The patient in this vignette presents with progression of his ALS as evidenced by increasing need for noninvasive ventilation support, as well as decreased oral intake. The patient is unable to participate in decisions as he is lethargic and does not have decision-making capacity. A goals-of-care discussion is held with the patient's mother, who is listed as the legal surrogate on his advance care planning document retrieved in the electronic health record. Review of the advance directive indicates that the patient would want a time-limited trial of ventilator and feeding tube. A meeting is held with his mother in the resuscitation room, as the patient is boarding in the ED hallway. The emergency physician asks the mother what she understands, to which the patient's mother cries and says, "He is getting worse." The emergency physician responds, "Yes, we are in a different place. Your son's ALS is worsening. I wish things were different." The emergency clinician and emergency nurse wait a few moments before proceeding, allowing the mother to cry softly. The emergency clinicians ask, "Based on your son's worsening inability to breathe due to his ALS, we are at the place of needing to consider if we will place a breathing tube that I feel will be permanent." Based on the patient's values as documented in his advance directive and what his mother states—he would want to be on the ventilator and have a feeding tube for some time if he could still communicate with his family through some means. Based on the discussion, the emergency physician proposes the plan to intubate in the ED and admit to the ICU with the plan for trial of a tracheostomy and feeding tube.

KEY POINTS

- Confirm that the necessary people are present for the meeting.
- Assess understanding of illness, make no assumptions.
- Ask permission to proceed throughout the conversation.
- Respond to emotion with empathy.
- Make recommendations based on values, and priorities identified.

Further Reading

1. Grudzen CR, Emlet LL, Kuntz J, et al. EM talk: Communication skills training for emergency medicine patients with serious illness. *BMJ Supportive & Palliative Care.* 2016;6:219–224.
2. Paladino J, Fromme EK. Preparing for serious illness: A model for better conversations over the continuum of care. *Am Fam Physician.* 2019;99(5):281–284.
3. https://pubmed.ncbi.nlm.nih.gov/30811166/?dopt=Abstract
4. Vital talk. http://www.vitaltalk.org
5. Back A, Arnold R, Tulsky J. *Mastering communication with seriously ill patients.* Cambridge University Press; 2009.
6. Weissman DE. Decision making at a time of crisis near the end of life. *JAMA.* 2004;292:1738–1743.
7. Hudson P, Quinn K, O'Hanlon B, Aranda S. Family meetings in palliative care: Multidisciplinary clinical practice guidelines. *BMC Palliat Care.* 2008;7:12.

8. Lautrette A, Ciroldi M, Ksibi H, Azoulay E. End-of-life family conferences: Rooted in the evidence. *Crit Care Med.* 2006;34(11 Suppl):S364–S372.

9. Weissman DE, Quill TE, Arnold RM. Preparing for the family meeting #222. *J Palliat Med.* 2010 Feb;13(2):203–204; Weissman DE, Quill TE, Arnold RM. The family meeting: starting the conversation #223. *J Palliat Med.* 2010 Feb;13(2):204–205; Weissman DE, Quill TE, Arnold RM. Responding to emotion in family meetings #224. *J Palliat Med.* 2010 Mar;13(3):327–328; Weissman DE, Quill TE, Arnold RM. The family meeting: causes of conflict #225. *J Palliat Med.* 2010 Mar;13(3):328–329; Weissman DE, Quill TE, Arnold RM. Helping surrogates make decisions #226. *J Palliat Med.* 2010 Apr;13(4):461–462; Weissman DE, Quill TE, Arnold RM. The family meeting: end-of-life goal setting and future planning #227. *J Palliat Med.* 2010 Apr;13(4):462–463.

10. Bernacki R, Hutchings M, Vick J, Smith G, Paladino J, Lipsitz S, et al. Development of the Serious Illness Care Program: A randomised controlled trial of a palliative care communication intervention. *BMJ Open.* 2015;5(10):e009032.

11. Geerse OP, Lamas DJ, Sanders JJ, Paladino J, Kavanagh J, Henrich NJ, et al. A qualitative study of serious illness conversations in patients with advanced cancer. *J Palliat Med.* 2019;22(7):773–781.

12. Childers JW, Back AL, Tulsky JA, Arnold, RM. REMAP: A framework for goals of care conversations. *J Oncol Pract.* 2017;13(10):e844–e850.

4 "Read the Papers, Please"

Alina M. Fomovska and Eric Isaacs

Case: A 68-year-old male with end-stage renal disease and metastatic lung cancer with brain metastasis presents to the emergency department (ED) with fever, hypotension, and altered mental status. The patient last had dialysis one day prior to ED presentation. His wife is present at bedside and says that she has noticed him getting worse over the last few days and was unsure how to help him. On examination, you determine that the patient does not have decision-making capacity. The patient has an advance directive in the electronic medical record that says that if he had a terminal condition, he would want his natural death to occur and names his wife as the legal surrogate. In the course of discussion, you ask the wife about continuation dialysis and other life-sustaining interventions, and she says she feels he would "definitely" want to continue dialysis and would want a trial of intubation.

What do you do now?

ADVANCE DIRECTIVES IN THE EMERGENCY DEPARTMENT

This is a difficult situation that can be a cause of moral distress for providers. Some may dread the clinical situation described above: the stakes are high, and there is a burden to doing the morally "right" thing. As emergency providers, much of the moral distress comes from feeling like we are doing the "wrong" thing. When treating a patient who is likely at the end of life, pursuing aggressive and invasive interventions with the potential to inflict suffering may compound that feeling. This is especially true when the patient has expressed wishes seeming contrary to the actions requested by family. For the sake of consistency and brevity, throughout this discussion we use the term "family" to refer to the individuals surrounding the patient who are involved in their care and who may be acting as chosen or surrogate decision makers. We use the term to convey a sense of closeness, rather than blood relation. Over time, these experiences build in the psyche and can be a significant contributor to provider burnout. A hallmark of emergency medicine practice is the imperative to make high-stakes decisions, with limited information, under tight time constraints. This is especially evident when faced with resuscitating a critically ill patient, who cannot speak for themselves, with a range of possible life-sustaining interventions that could be employed. Advance directives—written documents communicating a patient's provisional wishes for care—can help guide the team in providing care that is most in line with the patient's goals. Advance care planning documents typically have two functions: (1) the ability to appoint a legal surrogate decision maker and (2) the ability to express the patient's wishes for life-sustaining therapy should they have a terminal condition. In addition to written documentation, we rely on the surrogate's interpretation of the care the patient would have wanted to receive were they able to express their desires. At times, however, these sources of direction may feel at odds with one another. Having a series of tools to approach care at the end of life empowers emergency providers to navigate emotionally and ethically difficult conversations, provide the best possible care, and leave a shift with a lighter conscience.

When caring for an individual at the end of life, the physician's responsibility is primarily to the patient but also includes the family. Our primary duty, first and foremost, is to the patient. However, when caring for patients at the end of life, providers may feel like they are being acted on by contradictory forces. In caring for those with serious illness, the definition of "patient" expands beyond the individual in the gurney and begins to include the surrounding family. Our interventions can have a profound impact on the family for years even after the patient's death.

A family needs "a story they can live with." This may mean different things (e.g., "I did not give up on my loved one" or "I made sure they did not suffer"). Emergency providers can skillfully navigate and frame situations appropriately, moderating expectations of both the family and the medical team, and compromise on treatment plans. Including the family within the sphere of patient care allows discussions about advance directives and goals of care to shift from a potentially contentious topic to a therapeutic one. One important role of the medical provider is to share the burden of end-of-life decision-making by interpreting the clinical situation and offering a recommendation in the context of patient values. This is a difficult task, as providers may feel ill-equipped to provide a recommendation, or they may feel that doing so would be an encroachment of the family's autonomy. Resuscitative procedures, however, are medical interventions, and family members deserve our interpretation of the clinical situation and treatment options. A provider's recommendation may also play a big role in alleviating the guilt or distress that families feel pursuing a difficult end-of-life decision, allowing the conversation to focus on the patient's wishes.

There are a variety of advance directives that may be encountered in the ED (Table 4.1). Advance directives are legal documents that exist in every state. States vary in specific documentation requirements, subjects covered, and legal scope (including whether a patient's documented decisions can be overridden by family when the patient loses decision-making capacity). It is important to know how the laws apply in your state. There are three general types of advance directives.

1. *Healthcare power of attorney.* Also known as a "healthcare proxy form" or "healthcare agent form," this document allows a patient to indicate an agent to make healthcare-related decisions in the event they are unable to do so. In the absence of power of attorney documentation, decision-making responsibility falls to surrogate decision makers according to state-specific statutory priority lists. States vary in the priority order that family members appear, and

TABLE 4.1 **Advance Directives**

Document	"Also Known As"	Purpose	Notes
Healthcare power of attorney	Healthcare proxy form Healthcare agent form	Allows a patient to indicate an agent to make healthcare-related decisions in the event they are unable to do so.	In the absence of power of attorney documentation, decision-making responsibility falls to surrogate decision makers according to state-specific statutory priority lists.
Living will	Healthcare directive	Written description of the patient's wishes regarding medical treatment (may provide the greatest detail about patient values and preferences).	Not signed by a physician. In many states these documents are not legally binding.
POLST form (Physician Orders for Life Sustaining Treatment)	POST (Physician Orders for Scope of Treatment) MOLST (Medical Orders for Life-Sustaining Treatment) MOST (Medical Orders for Scope of Treatment)	Translates the wishes expressed in an advance directive to medical orders.	Brightly colored, portable, paper form signed by a physician with orders pertaining to treatments at the end of life.

whether common-law spouses or friends are included. Some states do not have an established hierarchy of surrogate decision makers. Notably, a *healthcare* power of attorney differs from a *financial* power of attorney, and a document granting an individual power over financial matters should not be interpreted as extending to medical decisions.

2. *Living will.* Also known as a "healthcare directive," this document is a written description of the patient's wishes regarding medical treatment. Living wills are not signed by a physician and in many states are not legally binding, but they may provide the greatest detail about patient values and preferences.

3. *POLST form ("Physician Orders for Life-Sustaining Treatment).* In some states referred to as the POST (Physician Orders for Scope of Treatment), MOLST (Medical Orders for Life-Sustaining Treatment), or MOST (Medical Orders for Scope of Treatment). This document translates the wishes expressed in an advance directive to medical orders. This is often a brightly colored, portable, paper form signed by a physician with orders pertaining to treatments at the end of life. It typically covers CPR and intubation preferences, the focus of treatment (comfort vs. limited interventions vs. full treatment), and acceptability of artificial nutrition. States vary in whether surrogate decision makers may override preferences indicated personally by the patient (Figure 4.1).

Some patients may have a nontraditional expression of their end-of-life wishes. This includes items such as tattoos, medallions, and bracelets. These are not legal documents, and their interpretation requires extreme caution. Given the lack of standardization, nontraditional directives cannot be reliably interpreted and should not be relied upon to determine medical courses of action. Limited research on this topic demonstrates that patients may obtain and display nontraditional directives for a variety of reasons—to commemorate an important event, communicate an overall philosophy or idea, or be considered in very specific circumstances. Nontraditional advance directives may be used to help understand a patient's values, but they should not take priority over standard care and practice—such as attempting to stabilize a patient to allow them to resume decisional capacity, locating standard advance directives, or relying on surrogate decision makers.

Advance directives are never sufficiently nuanced to cover each clinical scenario a patient faces. Given their limitations, how do we make use of these documents? It would not be reasonable to expect a patient to predict every possible medical situation and delineate their preferred course of

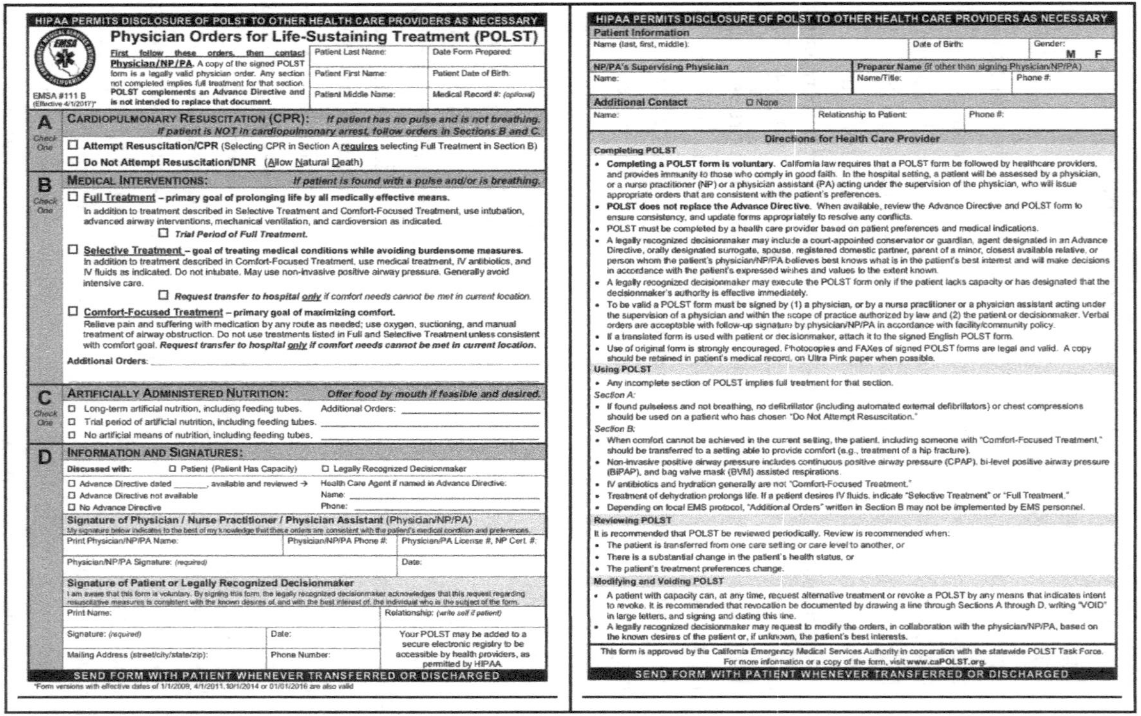

HIPAA PERMITS DISCLOSURE OF POLST TO OTHER HEALTH CARE PROVIDERS AS NECESSARY

Physician Orders for Life-Sustaining Treatment (POLST)

EMSA #111 B (Effective 4/1/2017)*

First follow these orders, then contact Physician/NP/PA. A copy of the signed POLST form is a legally valid physician order. Any section not completed implies full treatment for that section. **POLST complements an Advance Directive and is not intended to replace that document.**

Patient Last Name:	Date Form Prepared:
Patient First Name:	Patient Date of Birth:
Patient Middle Name:	Medical Record #: (optional)

A Check One — **CARDIOPULMONARY RESUSCITATION (CPR):** *If patient has no pulse and is not breathing. If patient is NOT in cardiopulmonary arrest, follow orders in Sections B and C.*

☐ **Attempt Resuscitation/CPR** (Selecting CPR in Section A requires selecting Full Treatment in Section B)

☐ **Do Not Attempt Resuscitation/DNR** (Allow Natural Death)

B Check One — **MEDICAL INTERVENTIONS:** *If patient is found with a pulse and/or is breathing.*

☐ **Full Treatment – primary goal of prolonging life by all medically effective means.** In addition to treatment described in Selective Treatment and Comfort-Focused Treatment, use intubation, advanced airway interventions, mechanical ventilation, and cardioversion as indicated.

☐ ***Trial Period of Full Treatment.***

☐ **Selective Treatment – goal of treating medical conditions while avoiding burdensome measures.** In addition to treatment described in Comfort-Focused Treatment, use medical treatment, IV antibiotics, and IV fluids as indicated. Do not intubate. May use non-invasive positive airway pressure. Generally avoid intensive care.

☐ ***Request transfer to hospital only** if comfort needs cannot be met in current location.*

☐ **Comfort-Focused Treatment – primary goal of maximizing comfort.** Relieve pain and suffering with medication by any route as needed; use oxygen, suctioning, and manual treatment of airway obstruction. Do not use treatments listed in Full and Selective Treatment unless consistent with comfort goal. ***Request transfer to hospital only if comfort needs cannot be met in current location.***

Additional Orders: ____________

C Check One — **ARTIFICIALLY ADMINISTERED NUTRITION:** *Offer food by mouth if feasible and desired.*

☐ Long-term artificial nutrition, including feeding tubes. Additional Orders: ____________

☐ Trial period of artificial nutrition, including feeding tubes.

☐ No artificial means of nutrition, including feeding tubes.

D — **INFORMATION AND SIGNATURES:**

Discussed with: ☐ Patient (Patient Has Capacity) ☐ Legally Recognized Decisionmaker

☐ Advance Directive dated ______, available and reviewed → Health Care Agent if named in Advance Directive:
☐ Advance Directive not available — Name:
☐ No Advance Directive — Phone:

Signature of Physician / Nurse Practitioner / Physician Assistant (Physician/NP/PA)
My signature below indicates to the best of my knowledge that these orders are consistent with the patient's medical condition and preferences.

Print Physician/NP/PA Name:	Physician/NP/PA Phone #:	Physician/PA License #, NP Cert. #:
Physician/NP/PA Signature: (required)		Date:

Signature of Patient or Legally Recognized Decisionmaker
I am aware that this form is voluntary. By signing this form, the legally recognized decisionmaker acknowledges that this request regarding resuscitative measures is consistent with the known desires of, and with the best interest of, the individual who is the subject of the form.

Print Name:		Relationship: (write self if patient)
Signature: (required)	Date:	Your POLST may be added to a secure electronic registry to be accessible by health providers, as permitted by HIPAA.
Mailing Address (street/city/state/zip):	Phone Number:	

SEND FORM WITH PATIENT WHENEVER TRANSFERRED OR DISCHARGED

*Form versions with effective dates of 1/1/2009, 4/1/2011, 10/1/2014 or 01/01/2016 are also valid

HIPAA PERMITS DISCLOSURE OF POLST TO OTHER HEALTH CARE PROVIDERS AS NECESSARY

Patient Information

Name (last, first, middle):	Date of Birth:	Gender: M F

NP/PA's Supervising Physician	**Preparer Name** (if other than signing Physician/NP/PA)	
Name:	Name/Title:	Phone #:

Additional Contact ☐ None		
Name:	Relationship to Patient:	Phone #:

Directions for Health Care Provider

Completing POLST

- **Completing a POLST form is voluntary.** California law requires that a POLST form be followed by healthcare providers, and provides immunity to those who comply in good faith. In the hospital setting, a patient will be assessed by a physician, or a nurse practitioner (NP) or a physician assistant (PA) acting under the supervision of the physician, who will issue appropriate orders that are consistent with the patient's preferences.
- **POLST does not replace the Advance Directive.** When available, review the Advance Directive and POLST form to ensure consistency, and update forms appropriately to resolve any conflicts.
- POLST must be completed by a health care provider based on patient preferences and medical indications.
- A legally recognized decisionmaker may include a court-appointed conservator or guardian, agent designated in an Advance Directive, orally designated surrogate, spouse, registered domestic partner, parent of a minor, closest available relative, or person whom the patient's physician/NP/PA believes best knows what is in the patient's best interest and will make decisions in accordance with the patient's expressed wishes and values to the extent known.
- A legally recognized decisionmaker may execute the POLST form only if the patient lacks capacity or has designated that the decisionmaker's authority is effective immediately.
- To be valid a POLST form must be signed by (1) a physician, or by a nurse practitioner or a physician assistant acting under the supervision of a physician and within the scope of practice authorized by law and (2) the patient or decisionmaker. Verbal orders are acceptable with follow-up signature by physician/NP/PA in accordance with facility/community policy.
- If a translated form is used with patient or decisionmaker, attach it to the signed English POLST form.
- Use of original form is strongly encouraged. Photocopies and FAXes of signed POLST forms are legal and valid. A copy should be retained in patient's medical record, on Ultra Pink paper when possible.

Using POLST

- Any incomplete section of POLST implies full treatment for that section.

Section A:

- If found pulseless and not breathing, no defibrillator (including automated external defibrillators) or chest compressions should be used on a patient who has chosen "Do Not Attempt Resuscitation."

Section B:

- When comfort cannot be achieved in the current setting, the patient, including someone with "Comfort-Focused Treatment," should be transferred to a setting able to provide comfort (e.g., treatment of a hip fracture).
- Non-invasive positive airway pressure includes continuous positive airway pressure (CPAP), bi-level positive airway pressure (BiPAP), and bag valve mask (BVM) assisted respirations.
- IV antibiotics and hydration generally are not "Comfort-Focused Treatment."
- Treatment of dehydration prolongs life. If a patient desires IV fluids, indicate "Selective Treatment" or "Full Treatment."
- Depending on local EMS protocol, "Additional Orders" written in Section B may not be implemented by EMS personnel.

Reviewing POLST

It is recommended that POLST be reviewed periodically. Review is recommended when:

- The patient is transferred from one care setting or care level to another, or
- There is a substantial change in the patient's health status, or
- The patient's treatment preferences change.

Modifying and Voiding POLST

- A patient with capacity can, at any time, request alternative treatment or revoke a POLST by any means that indicates intent to revoke. It is recommended that revocation be documented by drawing a line through Sections A through D, writing "VOID" in large letters, and signing and dating this line.
- A legally recognized decisionmaker may request to modify the orders, in collaboration with the physician/NP/PA, based on the known desires of the patient or, if unknown, the patient's best interests.

This form is approved by the California Emergency Medical Services Authority in cooperation with the statewide POLST Task Force. For more information or a copy of the form, visit www.caPOLST.org.

SEND FORM WITH PATIENT WHENEVER TRANSFERRED OR DISCHARGED

FIGURE 4.1. State of California POLST form.

care. Therefore, advance directives typically represent general, and at times, frustratingly vague guidelines. In this case, the patient's advance directive indicates that "if he had a terminal condition, he would want his natural death to occur." But what does this actually mean? For some patients, this may reflect their preference only for the last days of life, and any and all life-sustaining intervention up to that point would be entirely acceptable. Other patients may choose to forego any life-prolonging treatment at the time of diagnosis with a terminal illness. Our patient's completed advance directives do not indicate where he falls on this spectrum.

An important role that advance directives play is that in completing them, patients have an opportunity to discuss values and wishes with their family. These conversations, unlike documentation forms, are able to reflect greater subtlety and may elucidate much greater nuance behind a box on the form. When presented with an existing advance directive, ask the surrogate decision makers what they have discussed with their loved one on this subject.

Requisite is an understanding of where the patient is in their disease trajectory. Diseases follow often-predictable trajectories to decline. Understanding these trajectories can aid the process of prognostication, which is crucial in considering when and how to apply advance directives.

1. *"Sudden death"* describes events such as massive hemorrhagic stroke or trauma. A patient is at a high functional level until a sudden event rapidly reduces their functional status.

2. *"Organ failure"* is a typical trajectory of diseases such as congestive heart failure or end-stage renal disease. Patients may start at a relatively high functional status and experience gradual decline, characterized by intermittent decompensations, with recovery that does not reach the previous health baseline. This might be described as a "roller coaster" experience.

3. *"Terminal illness"* depicts the course of many cancers. At the time of diagnosis, patients may be at a relatively high functional status and may remain so for a period of time with only a slow decline. Eventually, however, the decline becomes much more rapid and consistent toward death.

4. *"Frailty"* is a typical course for diseases such as dementia, with a relatively low initial functional status, and a very slow and gradual curve toward decline. Families may describe this as "a very long road."

Our patient is likely on the rapid downward slope of the "terminal illness" trajectory. He may also experience the decompensation and partial recovery that characterize "organ failure." Understanding his prognostic trajectory can help guide conversations about further decisions and interventions.

Given this likely presentation of sepsis, antibiotics and fluids may allow him to recover some functional status after this decompensation. While he is very unlikely to return to a pre-event baseline, he may be able to engage in a conversation with family and medical providers, and make concrete plans to address his wishes. Perhaps after a treatment course, he would be able to return home if that is within his wishes. In that case, more aggressive treatment at this point would actually help the patient achieve his overall goals for a natural and peaceful death.

The "Is this it?" moment. Most people say they would prefer a natural and peaceful death. However, when confronted with the questions of "code status," many choose those "aggressive interventions" seemingly contrary to that end. This tension can be summed as: "Everyone wants to die a natural and peaceful death—but not yet." In most cases, patients experience more and more medical interventions as they approach the end of life. Many are effective at prolonging the length, and sometimes the quality, of patients' lives. Until they no longer do. Patients and their families rely on their medical team to tell them when "this is it." It is a mistake to assume that families have accurately identified the terminal event. Understanding the medical situation and the patient's condition allows families to act more accurately in accordance to their loved one's wishes. If, in your clinical assessment, the patient is facing an event that will likely lead to their death, it is important to communicate this to their family directly. This allows the conversation to refocus from a general discussion to specific treatments that should be pursued at this time.

A "time-limited trial" is a powerful tool in end-of-life care. The resuscitation room may feel like an inopportune space to engage in conversations about end of life—conversations that ideally require ample time, rapport, and a deep understanding of the patient's clinical condition and social dynamic. These limitations, however, do not preclude the emergency provider from having a thoughtful and impactful interaction with family about appropriate courses of care. When the clinical situation is clear and the patient is imminently dying, it is imperative to inform the family and provide a recommendation based on the information available. When the case is less clear, or when family is not ready to defer life-prolonging interventions, a powerful tool is the concept of a "time-limited trial." To be effective, a provider introducing the concept of a time-limited trial needs to be clear about what the procedure entails, including the indication (e.g., clinical uncertainty, possibility of response to treatment, lack of time or resource to have an in-depth conversation with family about further steps of case, or to provide an opportunity for family to gather) and a set time expectation (usually a precise and limited time scope—e.g., 24 or 48 hours). With this intervention, families are prepared for further conversations and may begin processing the change in their loved one's clinical status. Do not underestimate the power of introducing a time-limited trial in the ED. A patient may still go up to the intensive care unit (ICU) intubated. However, when the emergency provider has discussed the intervention from the point of view of a "time-limited trial," the family may moderate expectations appropriately. If the patient's condition does not improve, the conversation that the ICU team initiates later takes on a profoundly different tone than if the idea of a time-limited trial had not been broached.

When conflicts arise between the emergency care team and the surrogate/family regarding the provision of care that is contrary to the patient's advance care planning document, the emergency clinician will need to decide in the moment what is best for the patient by weighing all the factors. If there is time, ethics and legal can be consulted.

In our case, what do you do in this situation, now? It is difficult to know if this is the patient's terminal event, or if his condition might be stabilized to a certain degree—perhaps allowing quality time with family or the opportunity to return home. Communicate your clinical assessment to the wife. If you suspect that his death is imminent, it is important to communicate that clearly. If you are uncertain, consider what the best or worst-case scenario may look like. Consider a statement like this:

"I know that this has been a really long journey for you both, and I can see what incredible care you have taken care of your husband. Based on what I am seeing today, I am worried that he is coming to the end of his life—and that this is the illness that is going to cause him to die. I'm very sorry." Allow silence. Address the discrepancy between what you have learned from the advance directives and what the wife has communicated. Consider a question such as:

"I can see that when your husband filled out his advance directive, he had indicated that if he were at the end of his life, he would want to experience a natural death. For most people, that usually means avoiding invasive treatments that prolong the dying process, such as being placed on a ventilator. Can you tell me more about conversations you have had about this?"

Don't be afraid to make a recommendation. In situations fraught with uncertainty, or when there may not be time for a detailed conversation, a time-limited trial may be the best option. Consider this statement:

"I'm very worried about your husband's breathing. From what I am hearing from you, it sounds like you two have discussed that, if this were to happen, it would be acceptable for him to be put on a ventilator for a short period of time, but that he would not want to be on the machine forever. We can put him on the ventilator now to see if his breathing improves. However, I am worried that despite what we do, he is going to die, and this treatment might hurt him more than help him. If his breathing does not get better in one or two days, my recommendation would be to respect his wishes and remove the breathing tube—and allow him to pass away naturally and peacefully. What do you think about that?"

CASE CONCLUSION

You have a conversation with the patient's wife as outlined above. After this discussion, his wife decides to agree to intubation at this time for a time-limited trial. The patient is intubated and started on broad-spectrum antibiotics. When the ICU team comes down to the ED to admit the patient, the patient's wife expresses her understanding of the situation. Together, the ICU team and the wife make a plan to reconvene after rounds tomorrow to determine whether the patient has benefited from a trial of intubation, and whether continuing the treatment would be in line with his values and wishes.

KEY POINTS

- At the end of life, our primary duty is to the patient. However, consider that our interventions can have a profound impact on the family for years to come; thus, it is important to include the family unit in your therapeutic consideration.
- Advance directives are legal documents that exist in every state. However, the extent different documents are legally binding, and whether or not family members can override the decisions expressed by the patient, varies from state to state. It is important to know the law where you practice.
- In cases of clinical ambiguity, or when family is not ready to defer life-prolonging interventions, a time-limited trial is a powerful tool that allows for further assessment of the patient while setting realistic expectations with the family.

Further Reading
1. Sabatino C. The evolution of health care advance planning law and policy. *Milbank Quarterly*. 2010;88(2):211–239.
2. DeMartino ES, Dudzinski DM, Cavan KD, Sperry BP, Gregory SE, Siegler M, Sylmasy DP, Mueller PS. Who decides when a patient can't? Statutes on alternate decision makers. *New England Journal of Medicine* 2017;376(15):1478–1482.
3. Goldish A, Rosielle D. Fast Facts and Concepts #365. Language for Routine Code Status Discussions. November 2018. https://www.mypcnow.org/fast-fact/langu age-for-routine-code-status-discussions/
4. Pollak KI, Childers JW, Arnold RM. Applying motivational interviewing techniques to palliative communication. *Journal of Palliative Medicine*. 2011;14(5):587–592.
5. Barclay JS, Blackhall LJ, Tulsky JA. Communication strategies and cultural issues in the delivery of bad news. *Journal of Palliative Medicine*. 2007;10(4):958–977.

6. Warm E, Rosielle D. Fast Facts and Concepts #12. Myths about Advance Directives. May 2018. https://www.mypcnow.org/fast-fact/myths-about-advance-directives/

7. "National POLST Program Designations." National POLST. https://polst.org/progr ams-in-your-state/?pro=1#top

8. Goldish A, Rosielle D. Fast Facts and Concepts #333. Recommending A Do Not Resuscitate Order for Patients with Advanced Illness. November 2018. https:// www.mypcnow.org/fast-fact/recommending-a-do-not-resuscitate-order-for-patie nts-with-advanced-illness/

9. Iverson KV. Nonstandard advance directives in emergency medicine: What should we do? *Journal of Emergency Medicine.* 2018 Jul;55(1):141–142.

10. Marco CA et al. Advance directives in emergency medicine: Patient perspectives and application to clinical scenarios. *American Journal of Emergency Medicine.* 2018;36(3):516–518.

11. Siddiqui S. A physician's moral dilemma in the emergency department: Going against a patient's perceived wishes. *Journal of Emergency Medicine.* 2016;51(6):748–749.

12. Grudzen CR, Buonocore P, Steinberg J, Ortiz JM, Richardson LD; AAHPM Research Committee Writing Group. Concordance of advance care plans with inpatient directives in the electronic medical record for older patients admitted from the emergency department. *Journal of Pain and Symptom Management.* 2016;51(4):647–651.

13. Song M, Ward SE. Disconnect between emergency contacts and surrogate decision-makers in the absence of advance directives. *Palliative Medicine.* 2014;27(8):789–792.

14. Escher M, Perrier A, Rudaz S, Dayer P, Perneger T. Doctors' decisions when faced with contradictory patient advance directives and health care proxy opinion: A randomized vignette-based study. *Journal of Pain and Symptom Management.* 2015;49(3):637–645.

5   I'm Suffocating

Daniel Bell

Case: A 22-year-old woman with advanced cystic fibrosis presents to the emergency department (ED) with severe shortness of breath. She reports a severe cough with green sputum and fever of 38.8 °C. In the ED, her vital signs are temperature of 39.0 °C, blood pressure of 125/75, heart rate of 120, respiratory rate of 32, and oxygen saturation of 92% on 2L nasal cannula. Her chest X-ray reveals left lower lobe infiltrate. Her white blood cell count is 24.5, and the rest of her labs are normal. She is not a candidate for transplant, though previously she has stated that she wished a trial of life-sustaining therapy should she worsen. In the ED, she is given antibiotics and is awaiting placement in the intensive care unit (ICU). Despite increasing supplemental oxygen and a saturation of 98%, the patient reports severe dyspnea and anxiety.

What do you do now?

DYSPNEA

This young woman is suffering from respiratory distress in advanced cystic fibrosis. Despite antibiotics and supplemental oxygen, she remains distressed by dyspnea. Dyspnea refers to the subjective feeling of breathlessness or breathing discomfort. The sensation of dyspnea may result from physiologic, psychological/emotional, spiritual, and/or environmental inputs. Our approach to dyspnea in this and other patients includes simultaneous symptom management while assessment and treatment of the underlying cause. When the underlying cause is not reversible, symptom management becomes the focus of our care.

Like the young woman in this vignette, it is common for patients with advanced illness to remain dyspneic despite initial efforts to treat underlying illness and correct vital sign abnormalities. Contributing factors for her dyspnea include (1) pneumonia and secretion burden that prevent optimal oxygen exchange through alveoli, creating a hypoxemia, which triggers increased respiratory drive via increased respiratory rate and tidal volume to maximize minute ventilation; (2) her sepsis (and work of breathing) is creating a metabolic acidosis, which drives her respiratory rate to compensate with respiratory alkalosis, to ventilate her acidemia as CO_2; (3) anxiety; and (4) not yet clearly identified psychological, social, or spiritual factors. In this patient, attending to symptom relief and facilitating a goals-of-care conversations about further treatment preferences can occur in the ED. Given her condition, discussion as to what we would do next if she were to deteriorate with hypoxia is prudent. She shares she would elect for a trial of ICU care. However, if knowing cystic fibrosis is an incurable illness that can lead to refractory respiratory failure, it would be appropriate to discuss preferences if medical interventions were unable to help her improve to breathe again on her own. Ideally, this conversation is done in a calm, supportive surrounding with caregiver support and known medical providers. However, given her situation, it is appropriate to broach this topic in the ED, ideally after improved symptom control, which will be outlined below. Discussion of noninvasive symptomatic/comfort-focused care, including hospice, should also be discussed as an option both at present or if intubated in the ICU without improvement.

CAUSES OF DYSPNEA

Physiologic

Dyspnea can refer to multiple distinct sensations and has several etiologies. However, generally it is thought to be rooted in either or both of the following: a "sensation" of air hunger mediated by chemoreceptors and mechanoreceptors signaling to the brainstem that something is wrong (such as hypoxia), or a "perception" of working hard to breathe mediated by signals from the brain to the pulmonary/motor system to fix the dilemma, particularly if the pulmonary/motor system cannot resolve the dilemma despite stronger signals, as may occur in bronchial constriction, muscle fatigue, hyperinflation, or pneumonia. Dyspnea occurs as result of awareness of activation in one or both arms of this feedback system, the afferent (signaling to the brain) or the efferent (signal from the brain to the respiratory system).

The stimulus for dyspnea in air hunger may be chemoreceptor mediated and/or mechanoreceptors mediated. Hypoxemia and hypercapnia are key drivers of dyspnea through triggering chemoreceptors in the carotid body and aortic arch. The medulla responds to pH and carbon dioxide only, and hypercapnia seems to be a much stronger trigger for dyspnea than hypoxia.

Mechanoreceptors in the airway, lungs, and chest wall sense alterations to flow, volume, and pressure of respiration. When pulmonary mechanics are disturbed in cases such as low flow (bronchoconstriction in asthma or anaphylaxis), low volume (pneumothorax), or high pressure (fibrosis), mechanoreceptors signal this dysfunction to the brain. Interestingly, as will be discussed later in "Therapeutics," mechanoreceptors in the face innervated by the trigeminal nerve can reduce sensation of dyspnea when triggered by flow of air, such as that created by a fan.

Through sensory feedback, the lungs and respiratory system maintain homeostasis in gas exchange (oxygenation) and acid-base balance (ventilation to adjust carbon dioxide levels to maintain normal pH). Hypoxia and hypercarbia can drive an increased rate of breathing, and at moderate levels our body may adjust without a sense of discomfort at all. At higher levels of physiologic disturbance, either/both the inciting factor (e.g., hypoxia) or the compensatory increased work of breathing may result in the sensation of dyspnea.

Psychological/Emotional

Anxiety, as our patient reports, is a common symptom in the setting of acute and chronic respiratory illness and is often present during an acute exacerbation. The cycle of breathlessness that includes fear and panic that induces a sensation of "doom" may accelerate respiratory rate that increases breathlessness in a vicious cycle. Emotional inputs affect experience of dyspnea. We know that perception of pain differs tremendously in varied emotional state: pain perception is likely to be augmented in times of fear, depression, loneliness, and attenuated in environments of personal inter-connectedness, empathy, and attention. Work on dyspnea is beginning to suggest a similar interconnected input. Studies have demonstrated that the perceived unpleasantness of shortness of breath episodes (dyspnea) is inde-pendent of simply how hard someone feels they are breathing; there can be more to triggering the sensation of unpleasantness or suffering than simply the physiologic input. Further, fear or worry about dyspnea based on past experiences significantly impacts experience of dyspnea, which interestingly can be attenuated with exposure therapy such as pulmonary rehabilitation. It is thus critical to attend to your patient's emotional state, respecting the influence it may exert on the patient's experience of suffering.

MANAGEMENT

See Table 5.1.

Pharmacological Measures

Oxygen is a medication with chemical and physiologic targets; it needs to be prescribed at an effective dose and can be toxic at high doses. Our patient is

TABLE 5.1 **Management of Dyspnea**

Pharmacological	Nonpharmacological	Advanced Respiratory Support
Oxygen	Fan	BIPAP
Opioids	Chaplains/RN support	HFNC
Benzodiazepines	Calm private space	Mechanical ventilation
	Mindfulness breathing	

benefitting from oxygen therapy with some relief, but not complete relief, of her dyspnea. Oxygen may be delivered with or without pressure; currently she is receiving oxygen via nasal cannula. For some patients, oxygenation with pressure palliates both chemoreceptor-mediated and/or mechanoreceptor-mediated dyspnea. While supplemental oxygenation alone is what helps some patients, the addition of a mechanical component may also help, as discussed later under "Advanced Respiratory Support." Of note, for people who are *not* hypoxic, oxygen supplies no greater relief in dyspnea than therapy with room air, allowing for consideration of less invasive means to improve airflow (such as a fan, described later in "Nonpharmacological Measures").

Opioids

Opioids are a valuable treatment option in soothing dyspnea. If done gently and incrementally, it is possible to provide relief and facilitate calmer, deeper breaths that maximize minute ventilation and improve compliance with ventilatory support, particularly when air trapping is of concern (in asthma, chronic obstructive pulmonary disease [COPD], and other obstructive pathologies). Opioids primarily work on dyspnea by targeting the central nervous system respiratory center in the brainstem, the medulla oblongata. This reduces the medulla's sensitivity to hypercarbia or hypoxia, decreasing sensation of dyspnea. The resultant decreased sensation of dyspnea typically allows for the patient to take deeper, fuller breaths, increasing the inspiratory: expiratory ratio and reduction in the overall respiratory rate without a rise in PCO_2 suggesting respiratory depression. A gentle trial of an IV opioid, such as an equianalgesic dose of morphine, fentanyl, or hydromorphone, may be advisable. The general rule is to go low and slow. Start with 1–2 mg IV morphine every 15 minutes until the patient reports lessening of the sensation of dyspnea.

Benzodiazepines

When the initiator of the anxiety is found to be breathlessness, it is important to treat the sensation of breathlessness first—hence the recommendation that opioids should be used before anxiolytics. The majority of studies in the use of benzodiazepines and dyspnea are in cancer and COPD patients. While some studies show harm and some show potential benefit, benzodiazepines may be considered as a second- or third-line treatment, when opioids and nonpharmacological measures have failed to control breathlessness. A Cochrane review did not demonstrate beneficial effect from benzodiazepine for the relief of dyspnea in people with advanced cancer or COPD. While they may provide anxiolysis, benzodiazepines may also cause sedation and increase risk of aspiration, respiratory suppression, and hypercarbia, and in some studies they have been shown to increase overall mortality. When considering the use of benzodiazepines, the lowest possible dose should be used after low-dose opioids have been tried.

Nonpharmacological Measures

Fan therapy is demonstrated to be effective in relieving dyspnea in patients with advanced cancer, postulated as a result of the relative lowering of facial surface temperature. This feeds back to the brainstem via mechanical receptors, as described earlier. Given the ease of use and zero adverse effects of this intervention, this finding should be extrapolated to use in other illness occurrences of dyspnea in the ED. A fan will not alter sensorium or impact communication, and it is a very reasonable first-line or adjuvant therapy.

For people without hypoxia, room air is as effective as oxygen in relieving dyspnea through nasal cannula. The mechanism hypothesized stimulates the trigeminal nerve, which feeds back to mechanical receptors similarly to room air above. This is a good reminder that without hypoxia, further up titrating wall oxygen is more likely to result in a nosebleed than improved dyspnea—it is time to reach for another tool.

Pay attention to surroundings. Providing a calm, quiet, monitored area can soothe the environmental inputs to dyspnea. Limit distraction and beeps/alarms to the extent possible. Slow, mindful breathing patterns can be encouraged by supportive staff. A chaplain can assist with spiritual or existential worries. Bedside nurses can monitor response to both medical and nonpharmacological calming therapies and work with patients on identifying and advocating for which approaches feel most helpful.

Advanced Respiratory Support

Advanced respiratory supportive therapies for dyspnea and/or to maintain oxygenation include noninvasive ventilation (bilevel positive airway pressure [BIPAP]), supplemental high-flow nasal cannula, and intubation with mechanical ventilation.

BIPAP has been established longer in adult populations, and it has been shown to improve mortality and decrease intubation in specific disease pathologies, namely cardiogenic pulmonary edema, COPD complicated by hypercarbia, and acute hypoxemic respiratory failure (which our patient currently has). The benefits of BIPAP are that it supports oxygenation, ventilation, provides positive end-expiratory pressure (PEEP), and can ease work of breathing. Downsides are typically related to the tightly fitted mask: it can be claustrophobic; it doesn't allow for secretion management/cough, eating, or drinking (dry mouth is a common complaint); and makes communication very difficult (cannot talk). BIPAP is not ideal in our patient's case: she would benefit from being able to speak and cough up secretions as they are loosened.

A second option is high flow nasal cannula (HFNC). HFNC is able to deliver high flows of heated and humidified oxygen with a precise level of fraction of inspired oxygen (FiO_2). Benefits include delivery of oxygen that is flowing at higher rates is easier to humidify and heat; thus, the improved humidification increases water content in secretions, allowing for more easily cleared mucous and decreased work of breathing. Downsides are that it is not a closed circuit thus cannot provide the PEEP or decreased work of breathing to the level that BIPAP can.

Finally, intubation and mechanical ventilation represent the highest level of invasive therapy. Benefits include maximal ability to deliver oxygenation and pressure support tailored to the patient's condition; it allows for bronchoscopy, aggressive pulmonary toilet, and decreased work of breathing. Downsides are that patients generally require sedation, cannot communicate, and in this case there is reason to believe once intubated she will either require a tracheostomy to continue long-term ventilation or transition to comfort care. Thus, for some patients this is goal discordant and may not be indicated.

Heliox is not commonly recommended or supported in the literature for general approach to dyspnea.

CASE CONCLUSION

For the patient in this vignette, based on prior informed conversations with her pulmonologist and family, she expressed her goals to have her pneumonia treated, and to do everything she could to make it back home, including a trial of mechanical ventilation if needed, but did not want to live on life support indefinitely. After one dose of 2 mg IV morphine, she reported feeling better and was able to talk, cough, and expectorate secretions. The respiratory therapist noted improved inspiratory:expiratory ratio, allowing for more effective gas exchange. One hour into her ED course, she experienced rapid worsening of oxygenation with a noted saturation of 85% on non-rebreather. A trial of HFNC was started along with a second dose of 2 mg IV morphine. After initiation of HFNC and the second dose of morphine, she was moved from the resuscitation room to a standard ED room, where a bedside fan was also used. Spiritual support services were consulted to assist with her anxiety, and she was able to express her deep fears of dying and, while tearful, expressed feeling better after being able to share her fears. Patient was admitted to the ICU and subsequently discharged 10 days later without need for mechanical ventilation.

KEY POINTS

- Opioids can assist with dyspnea synergistically with other disease-focused therapies.
- Benzodiazepines should be used with caution due to complications, and they do not have a significant evidence base.
- Use of HFNC can relieve breathlessness and assist in avoiding intubation.
- Nonpharmacological therapies such as fans have meaningful benefit in relieving dyspnea.

Further Reading

1. Abernethy AP, McDonald CF, Frith PA, et al. Effect of palliative oxygen versus room air in relief of breathlessness in patients with refractory dyspnea: A double-blind, randomised controlled trial. *Lancet.* 2010;376(9743):784–793. doi:10.1016/S0140-6736(10)61115-4. PMID: 20816546; PMCID: PMC2962424.
2. Kamal AH, Maguire JM, Wheeler JL, et al. Dyspnea review for the palliative care professional: Treatment goals and therapeutic options. *J Palliat Med.* 2012;15(1):106–114. doi:10.1089/jpm.2011.0110.

3. Parshall MB, Schwartzstein RM, Adams L, Banzett RB, Manning HL, Bourbeau J, Calverley PM, Gift AG, Harver A, Lareau SC, Mahler DA, Meek PM, O'Donnell DE; American Thoracic Society Committee on Dyspnea. An official American Thoracic Society statement: Update on the mechanisms, assessment, and management of dyspnea. *Am J Respir Crit Care Med.* 2012 Feb 15;185(4):435–452.

4. Simon ST, Higginson IJ, Booth S, et al. Benzodiazepines for the relief of breathlessness in advanced malignant and non-malignant diseases in adults. *Cochrane Database Syst Rev.* 2016;10(10):CD007354. doi:10.1002/14651858. CD007354.pub3

5. Kako J, Morita T, Yamaguchi T, et al. Fan therapy is effective in relieving dyspnea in patients with terminally ill cancer: A parallel-arm, randomized controlled trial. *J Pain Symptom Manage.* 2018;56(4):493–500. doi:10.1016/j.jpainsymman.2018.07.001

6. Banzett RB, Pedersen SH, Schwartzstein RM, Lansing RW. The affective dimension of laboratory dyspnea: Air hunger is more unpleasant than work/effort. *Am J Respir Crit Care Med.* 2008;177(12):1384–1390.

7. Janssens T, De Peuter S, Stans L, et al. Dyspnea perception in COPD: Association between anxiety, dyspnea-related fear, and dyspnea in a pulmonary rehabilitation program. *Chest.* 2011;140(3):618–625.

8. Azoulay E, Lemiale V, Mokart D, et al. Effect of high-flow nasal oxygen vs standard oxygen on 28-day mortality in immunocompromised patients with acute respiratory failure: The HIGH randomized clinical trial. *JAMA.* 2018;320(20):2099–2107. doi:10.1001/jama.2018.14282. PubMed PMID: 30357270; PubMed Central PMCID: PMC6583581.

9. Bernacki RE, Block SD. American College of Physicians High Value Care Task Force. Communication about serious illness care goals: A review and synthesis of best practices. *JAMA Intern Med.* 2014;174(12):1994–2003. doi:10.1001/jamainternmed.2014.5271. Review. PubMed PMID: 25330167.

10. Chmiel JF, Konstan MW. Inflammation and anti-inflammatory therapies for cystic fibrosis. *Clin Chest Med.* 2007;28(2):331–346. Review. PubMed PMID: 17467552.

11. Frat JP, Thille AW, Mercat A, et al. FLORALI Study Group; REVA Network. High-flow oxygen through nasal cannula in acute hypoxemic respiratory failure. *N Engl J Med.* 2015;372(23):2185–2196. doi:10.1056/NEJMoa1503326. Epub 2015 May 17. PubMed PMID: 25981908.

12. Madden BP, Kariyawasam H, Siddiqi AJ, et al. Noninvasive ventilation in cystic fibrosis patients with acute or chronic respiratory failure. *Eur Respir J.* 2002;19(2):310–313. Erratum in: *Eur Respir J.* 2002 Sep;20(3):790. PubMed PMID: 11866011.

13. Puntillo K, Nelson JE, Weissman D, et al. Advisory Board of the Improving Palliative Care in the ICU (IPAL-ICU) Project. Palliative care in the ICU: Relief of pain, dyspnea, and thirst—A report from the IPAL-ICU Advisory Board. *Intensive*

Care Med. 2014 Feb;40(2):235–248. doi:10.1007/s00134-013-3153-z. Review. PubMed PMID: 24275901; PubMed Central PMCID: PMC5428539.

14. Ward JJ. High-flow oxygen administration by nasal cannula for adult and perinatal patients. *Respir Care*. 2013;58(1):98–122. doi:10.4187/respcare.01941. Review. PubMed PMID: 23271822.

6 Make It Stop

Kate Aberger

Case: A 48-year-old woman with metastatic ovarian cancer presents to the emergency department (ED) with severe nausea and vomiting 5 days after chemotherapy. She reports that she is taking ondansetron 4 mg every 6 hours without relief. In the ED, she has a temperature of 37.0 °C, heart rate of 120 beats per minute, blood pressure of 102/60 mmHg, and a respiratory rate of 20 breaths per minute. Laboratory analysis reveals serum sodium of 148 mEq/L, chloride of 98 mEq/L, potassium of 4.5 mEq/L, carbon dioxide of 15 mEq/L, BUN of 32 mg/dL and creatinine of 1.2 mg/dL. On physical examination, her mucous membranes are dry. As you take the history, she reports that she is a mother of two; her children are 12 and 14 years old. She has been "fighting" this for 3 years. She reports that she has been taking chemotherapy now for that entire time and doesn't know why this last treatment has been so hard. She is worried about her family. She loves her oncologist, who has told her that they will not give up yet. She reports that she has been taking ondansetron for the last 5 days, and it just isn't helping. She reports that she doesn't have much nausea, mostly just vomiting everything she ingests. While taking the history, she begins to actively vomit.

What do you do now?

NAUSEA AND VOMITING

Nausea and vomiting are nonspecific symptoms with multiple etiologies.[1,2] Urgent and emergent causes of nausea and vomiting that signal disease exacerbation or progression in advanced cancer patients include hypercalcemia, malignant bowel obstruction, and increased intercranial pressure.[3,4,5] In patients with no history of cancer, causes such as uremia (in acute or chronic renal disease) and edema of the gastrointestinal tract (in acute or chronic heart failure) should be considered etiologies.[5,6] There are many common and less urgent causes that cause significant symptom burden without obvious etiology.[7] Urgent attention to the symptom management while etiologies are sought will decrease distress of patient and family while they are under our care.

This young woman is in obvious need of immediate symptom relief. A working differential for her nausea and vomiting is extensive. The differential includes chemotherapy-induced nausea and vomiting (CINV), bowel obstruction, new or worsening brain or liver metastasis, constipation, and gastritis/gastroparesis. There are some common causes of nausea and vomiting in advanced cancer (Table 6.1).[4,5,8] Each cause has a different pathophysiology and therefore a different treatment. In most cases there is overlap in cause and effective drugs.

At first glance, this woman has refractory nausea and vomiting due to chemotherapy. Could there be something else underlying? We need to think of other serious causes of nausea and vomiting in the setting of advanced cancer, including disease progression. Malignant bowel obstruction is also high on the differential, as any tumor burden in the abdomen can lead to compression or adhesion of bowel and lead to obstruction. While managing her symptoms, you order a computer tomography (CT) of her abdomen and pelvis to further evaluate if disease progression or obstruction exists. She is dehydrated as assessed on physical examination and verified by laboratory work: she has an anion gap metabolic acidosis—likely a lactic acidosis. A first-line intervention for symptom relief could be intravenous fluids. Typical symptoms of lactic acidosis may include nausea and vomiting, abdominal pain, weakness, tachycardia, and mental status changes.

For further symptom relief in addition to fluids, the mainstay in the emergency setting is pharmacological management. In this case, she has

TABLE 6.1 **Common Symptoms and Signs of Nausea and Vomiting in Patients with Cancer**

Symptoms	Etiology
Gastrointestinal	
Mouth pain/sores	Oropharyngeal infection (i.e., thrush/viral) esophagitis
Large high-volume emesis	High-level obstruction
Hematemesis	Varices perforated ulcer/mass
Excessive cough	Cough → increased abdominal pressure and nausea Pulmonary process → infection
Right-sided abdominal pain Colic	Liver, gallbladder disease
Constipation/obstipation	Constipation-related emesis, gastroparesis
Poor oral intake, cachexia	Anorexia
Increased abdominal girth, palpable masses, small-volume emesis	Squashed stomach syndrome from mass effect, ascites, small bowel obstruction
Metabolic	
Abdominal discomfort, confusion, kidney stones	Hypercalcemia
Decreased urine output, confusion	Renal failure
Labile blood pressure, syncopal episodes	Adrenal insufficiency
Confusion, changes in volume status	Hyponatremia
Neurologic	
Headaches, diplopia, early morning emesis, cranial nerve abnormalities	Increased intracranial pressure
Anxiety/nervousness	Anxiety-induced nausea

Adapted from Dietrich B, Ramchandran K, Von Roenn J. Nausea and vomiting. In: Jimmie C. Holland, William S. Breitbart, Paul B. Jacobsen, Matthew J. Loscalzo, Ruth McCorkle, Phyllis N. Butow, eds. *Psycho-oncology.* Oxford University Press; 2015:200.

already used ondansetron and failed. In order to choose the appropriate next intervention, we will review the emetogenic pathways as well as the pharmacology of the drugs that mitigate these pathways.

While nausea and vomiting have a complex pathophysiology that is still not fully understood, there are some commonly accepted mechanisms regarding the central mediation of nausea and vomiting.[8,9] Nausea and its resultant vomiting are controlled by (1) two areas in the medullary area of the brain, (2) the cerebral cortex, (3) the inner ear/vestibular system, and (4) the cerebellum with the resultant afferent effect of retching and vomiting. The medullary centers are the vomiting center and the chemoreceptor trigger zone (in the area postrema) and are both located in the medulla oblongata. The vomiting center receives input from the gut sensory receptors that are stimulated by gut distention, inflammation, or infection. The chemoreceptor trigger zone (CTZ) is rich in various receptors to include histamine (H1), muscarinic, dopamine (D_2) and serotonin ($5HT_3$ and $5HT_4$), neurokinins (NK_1), and mu receptors. The CTZ lacks a specific blood-brain barrier and anatomically can detect emetogenic toxins in the blood as well as in the cerebrospinal fluid. The cerebral cortex receives input more globally. Metabolic disturbances (such as uremia, electrolyte imbalance, for example hypercalcemia or hyponatremia) can also stimulate the vomiting center. Other cortical stimulants include emotional, spiritual, and psychological inputs such as loss of personhood, grief, worry, anxiety, and fear. Cumulatively, these afferent stimuli result in the efferent stimulation of the vagal nerve, which results in the act of vomiting (Figure 6.1).[9]

Pharmacological therapies that block these receptors represent the foundational basis for the pharmacological management of nausea and vomiting (Table 6.2).[8] Pharmacological agent classes include serotonin antagonists, dopamine antagonists, histamine antagonists, anticholingeric agents, muscarinic antagonists, and neurokinin antagonists.[8,9,10] When using pharmacological agents, one should try and block multiple receptors with multiple medications of different classes. A common pharmacological strategy might be to begin with a serotonin antagonist followed by a dopamine antagonist, followed by an anticholinergic agent. While the mechanism is not quite understood, glucocorticoids can be very effective in the management of nausea and vomiting. Glucocorticoid receptors are noted to be

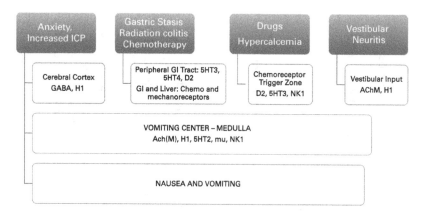

FIGURE 6.1. Pathophysiology of vomiting.

widespread in the brain that input to the vomiting center. Other agents include benzodiazepines, which are thought to work at the level of the cortex for a combination effect of sedation, anti-anxiety, and possibly depression of the vomiting center. Cannabinoids have their effect at the level of the enterochromaffin cells in the gastrointestinal tract and also have an anti-cholinergic effect on Auerbach's plexus and the prostaglandin cyclic nucleotide system. Typically, in combination with serotonin or dopamine antagonist, glucocorticoids can be very effective for nausea and vomiting for short periods of time. Nonpharmacological interventions are many include meditation, acupuncture, cognitive behavioral therapy, and spiritual support.

If chemotherapy is a contributor to the patient's nausea and vomiting, there are five historical factors to consider in relationship to chemotherapy[8-11]: (1) *Acute* occurs within 24 hours of chemotherapy; (2) *Delayed* occurs between 24 hours and 5 days; (3) *Breakthrough* occurs despite attempts to treat prophylactically; (4) *Anticipatory* occurs when triggered by taste, odor, memories, visions, or anxiety related to chemotherapy; and (5) *Refractory* occurs during subsequent cycles of chemotherapy without relief from antiemetics. There are numerous chemotherapeutic agents, each with their own potential to cause nausea and vomiting graded via their emetogenic potential incidence: high (>90%), medium (30%–90%), minimal (10%–30%), or low (<10%). For patients who receive high or medium emetogenic chemotherapy regimens—they will be prescribed

TABLE 6.2 **Pharmacological Management of Nausea and Vomiting**

Drug	Neurotransmitters/Mechanism	Side Effects/Issues	Dosing
Antipsychotic; dopamine antagonist	D2 antagonist	Extrapyramidal symptoms (EPS), sedation	Haloperidol: 0.5 mg–5 mg/dose q8h (SC/IV = ½ PO)
Antipsychotics	H1 antagonist, ACH antagonist, lessor D2 antagonist	EPS	Chlorpromazine: 0.5 mg–1 mg/kg q8h (IV = PO)
Promotility agent; dopamine antagonist	D2 antagonist, 5HT$_4$ agonist at gut	· Increases GI motility · Good for gastroparesis, bad for total mechanical obstruction	Metoclopramide: 5–15 mg before meals and bedtime (IV/SC = PO)
Antivertigo/antiemetic	· ACH-M1 antagonists · H1 antagonists	Anticholinergic side effects, likely bad choices in elderly, delirious, or cognitively impaired patients	· Scopolamine: 0.5 mg transdermal PATCH q3d · Meclizine: 25 mg TID
Serotonin receptor antagonist	5HT$_3$ antagonist	Costly	· Granisetron: 1 mg q12h · Ondansetron: 0.15 mg/kg/dose q6h (max. 8 mg/d)
Steroids	· Capillary permeability · Intracranial pressure · Edema, capsular stretch	Hypertension, gastritis, osteoporosis, myopathy, mood swings, hyperglycemia, immunosuppression, delirium	· Dexamethasone: 6–10 mg load, then 2–4 mg bid or qid for maintenance · Prednisone: 1.5 mg dexamethasone = 10 mg prednisone
Antihistamine	H1 antagonist	· Sedation · Can cause confusion in older adults	· Diphenhydramine: 1 mg/kg/dose PO q4h (max: 100 mg/dose) · Hydroxyzine: 0.5–1.0 mg/kg/dose q4h (max: 600 mg/day)
Somatostatin analogue		Costly	Octreotide: 50–100 micrograms subQ tid, can increase to 900 µg per day

Source: Hesketh PJ et al. Antiemetics: American Society of Clinical Oncology clinical practice guideline update. *Journal of Clinical Oncology.* 2017;35(28):3240–3262.

premedication regimens typically to include a serotonin antagonist and a dopamine antagonist +/– a glucocorticoid. For patients who present to the ED with recent or current chemotherapy administration, the clinician should inquire about any premedication regimens the patient was prescribed. Patients may not understand the significance of a premedication regimen and instead of using it in a scheduled fashion may only have been using it in an "as-needed" fashion.

Radiation therapy may also cause nausea and vomiting—radiation-induced nausea and vomiting (RINV). Release of histamines and other transmitters are thought to be the cause of RINV.[8] It has been shown that 5-hydroxytryptamine (5-HT) is released in response to the radiation and acts on the 5-HT receptor—a known receptor in the vomiting center. Hence, the first-line pharmacological agent in the prevention of RINV is a serotonin antagonist and should also be the first-line agent should a patient develop RINV followed by a dopamine antagonist. Like CINV, RINV prophylaxis, radiation regimens can be mild, moderate, or severe. Mild/low emetogenic potential regimens are typically to the head, neck, or extremities; moderate to the upper abdomen, neck, or cranium; or severe to the half or total body.

Other important considerations for assessment and management of nausea and vomiting include a focus on anything that can reduce distention of the gut, increase forward motility, and decrease bowel intraluminal or luminal distention. Gut distention and irritability promote signals to the vomiting center.[6-11] Hence, careful history of constipation or clinic suspicion of gastroparesis may signal the need to targeted therapy such as laxatives or prokinetic agents. When obstruction is a possible factor, prokinetic agents should not be used acutely. In the case of bowel wall edema as the cause, for example in patients with refractory end-stage heart failure, diuretics (if no contraindication) may be a helpful source control treatment while also treating with agents that act centrally.

CASE CONCLUSION

For the patient in this vignette, given she was already taking ondansetron, you decide to target another receptor. You choose a dopamine receptor antagonist of low-dose haloperidol while she undergoes abdominal imaging of

CT. Her CT scan shows a small bowel obstruction and significant advancement of her ovarian tumors. There is new metastasis to the peritoneum, causing partial obstruction with multiple dilated loops of small bowel. To decrease enteric distention, she receives a nasogastric tube with over 1000 cc of liquid return. Overall, she reports feeling much better. You consult surgical oncology for evaluation of her malignant small bowel obstruction as well as consult her oncologist. Her oncologist confides in you that she is worried her treatment options are becoming more limited.

When you talk with the patient again, you use more open-ended questions and listen actively and with the use of empathic statements. She confides that she is in quite a bit of pain at home, she is fatigued, and that she is nauseous all the time despite her home medications. She is struggling to maintain normality at home in front of her children and husband despite being extremely tired, in pain, and depressed. She cries when she is alone and now cries with you. You sit with her as she cries. When she is done, you acknowledge how much she is carrying and say, "This is really hard. I wish things were different." You tell her that with extra support, she can get her pain and other symptoms of nausea, vomiting, fatigue, and mood dysphoria under much better control in order to focus on what is most important. You suggest admission, and she agrees. You also recommend a consult with your palliative care colleagues while she is hospitalized this time. She states that she "doesn't want to give up," stating that "I'm not ready for hospice." You smile and gently educate her about what palliative care can offer—aggressive symptom management and support as she continues to pursue cancer-directed treatment. She visibly relaxes after she understands the difference between what you are offering and hospice. She is open to meeting with the palliative care service upon admission to continue symptom management, and social and psychological support.

Nausea and vomiting in the ED are common symptoms experienced by all patients, especially those with serious or life-limiting cancer and non-cancer illness.[12-14] A fundamental understanding of the pathophysiology of nausea and vomiting guides the pharmacological management of the symptoms. A clinical strategy that focuses on multiple receptor blockage is fundamental to the pharmacological management in the acute care setting.

- Do not delay immediate and aggressive pharmacological intervention while determining the underlying cause. Use receptor pharmacology to treat nausea and vomiting by targeting different pathways that contribute to symptoms.
- Determine and treat the underlying cause. Nausea and vomiting in advanced cancer have a unique differential, including malignant bowel obstruction, increased intracranial pressure, and hypercalcemia that need to be considered and tested for emergently. Adjust pharmacological interventions as cause becomes clear.
- Gentle goals-of-care discussions and compassionate communication are essential when discussing treatment options with patients with advanced cancer. More in-depth discussions regarding prognosis and aggressive treatment options like surgery may be necessary if patient has disease progression, is declining, or actively dying.
- Recommend palliative care follow-up or consult for further symptom management and further exploration of goals of care.

Further Reading

1. Quigley EMM, Hasler WL, Parkman HP. AGA technical review on nausea and vomiting. *Gastroenterology*. 2001;120:263–286.
2. Spiller RC. ABC of the upper gastrointestinal tract: Anorexia, nausea, vomiting, and pain. *BMJ*. 2001;323:1354–1357.
3. LeGrand SB. Nausea and vomiting in advanced cancer. *European Journal of Pharmacology*. 2014;722:187–191.
4. Harris DG. Nausea and vomiting in advanced cancer. *British Medical Bulletin*. 2010;96:175–185.
5. Tan A. Cancer emergencies. In: Quest A (ed.), *Palliative Aspects of Emergency Care*. Oxford American Palliative Care Library; 2013:23–36.
6. Collis E et al. Nausea and vomiting in palliative care. *BMJ*. 2015;3551:h6249.
7. Leach C. Nausea and vomiting in palliative care. *Clinical Medicine*. 2019;19(4):299–301.
8. Dietrich B, Ramchandran K, Von Roenn J. Nausea and vomiting. In: Emily Chai, Diane Meier, Jane Morris, Suzanne Goldhirsch, eds. *Psycho-oncology*. Oxford University Press; 2015.

9. Chai Q et al. Nausea and vomiting. In: Emily Chai, Diane Meier, Jane Morris, eds. *Geriatric Palliative Care: A Practical Guide for Clinicians*. Oxford University Press; 2014.

10. Hesketh PJ et al. Antiemetics: American Society of Clinical Oncology clinical practice guideline update. *Journal of Clinical Oncology*. 2017;35(28):3240–3262.

11. Walsh D et al. 2016 Updated MASCC/ESMO consensus recommendations: Management of nausea and vomiting in advanced cancer. *Support Care Cancer*. 2017;25(1):333–340.

12. Vandyk D et al. Emergency department visits for symptoms experienced by oncology patients: A systematic review. *Support Care Cancer*. 2012;20:11589–1599.

13. Sadik M et al. Attributes of cancer patients admitted to the emergency department in one year. *World Journal of Emergency Medicine*. 2014;5(2):85–90.

14. Delgado-Guay MO et al. Avoidable and unavoidable visits to the emergency department among patients with advanced cancer receiving outpatient palliative care. *Journal of Pain and Symptom Management*. 2015;49(3):497–504.

7 "I Would Rather Die"

Tammie E. Quest

Case: A 27-year-old male with metastatic osteosarcoma presents with progressive left leg pain from bony metastasis. At home he is taking morphine sustained-release 100 mg orally every 12 hours and oxycodone 20 mg every 4 hours around the clock. He presents to the emergency department (ED) for severe pain and is unable to walk due to pain. He reports that the pain is 10/10 in severity and is localized with a dull ache. He is unable to sleep due to the pain. Radiographs of the left femur show bony invasion of tumor without fracture. Laboratory studies are unremarkable.

What do you do now?

CANCER PAIN

Management of cancer pain includes assessment, knowledge of use of opioids and nonopioid strategies in the opioid-naive and opioid-tolerant patient, and an understanding of equianalgesic dosing, breakthrough pain dosing, and pharmacokinetics. The interdisciplinary team approach is critical in cancer pain management to attend to the physical, spiritual, psychological, and social aspects of a patients pain and can be initiated in the ED with the emergency department clinician, nurse, social worker, and chaplain all working together to ease suffering.

Cancer Pain Assessment

Assessment of cancer pain includes the characterization of the pain, the duration, location, and exacerbating factors of the pain. In advanced cancer, multiple cancer lesions may cause one or more of these pains in different areas. Pain may be classified as nociceptive (somatic or visceral), neuropathic, or mixed type (nociceptive pain + neuropathic). Pain can be characterized as somatic (pain located in the skin, muscles, ligaments, tendons, joints, or bones), visceral (located in an organ), or neuropathic (pain that invades or involves nerves). Somatic pain may be described as cramping, gnawing, aching, or sharp, and it can be localized; visceral pain may be described as deep squeezing, pressure, or aching in nature, and it cannot be well localized; neuropathic pain may be described as throbbing, hot or cold, tingling, stinging, electrical, pins and needles, numbness, or itching, and it may be localized, radiating, or diffuse. Due to the nature of solid tumor malignancy in particular, invasive lesions may cause one or all these types of pain. Numerical (0–10) and categorical (mild, moderate, severe) rating scales have shown to be an effective guide to measure the intensity and response to treatment in cancer pain.

Use of Opioids

Opioids are a first-line therapy for severe cancer pain in advanced cancer of all types. While it has been commonly thought that nociceptive pain is opioid responsive and neuropathic pain is not, studies have shown that in cancer pain, opioids can be effective in nociceptive, neuropathic, and mixed-pain cases. In patients who present to the ED, it is common that they are already taking opioids. In this case the emergency clinician must be facile in the evaluation and management of patients with severe cancer pain, including opioid dosing.

Nonopioid Strategies and Adjuvant Medications

For severe, uncontrolled cancer pain, a trial of opioids is the mainstay. Clinicians should be sure to look for acute reversible causes of pain such as urinary retention, relief of constipation, and relief of fluid collections (ascites, abscess, effusions). Adjuvant nonopioid therapies for cancer pain that may be helpful in the acute setting include nonsteroidal anti-inflammatory agents, steroids (to reduce inflammation), acetaminophen, and topical agents. When neuropathic pain exists, initiation of agents such as gabapentenoids and tricyclic antidepressants might be appropriate to initiate in the ED, though they may relieve pain over days versus minutes or hours.

Opioid Naive or Tolerant

When a decision has been made to use opioids, patients should be classified as opioid naive or opioid tolerant. Exquisitely careful history should be taken regarding how much opioid the patient has been taking on a regular basis. During the initial evaluation the clinician should determine if the patient is either opioid naive or opioid tolerant. Opioid tolerance is defined as greater than 60 oral morphine equivalents (OMEs) for 5 days. Tolerance in this context refers specifically to the patients' risk of toxicity from opioids. Patients who are tolerant are at decreased but not absent risk from opioid toxicity. Opioid toxicity is characterized in the early stages as neurologic toxicity that can be characterized by sedation, delirium, and pruritis, with the last side effect being respiratory depression. As patients take opioids on a regular basis, side effects will typically wane. Gastrointestinal side effects include nausea, vomiting, and constipation. Constipation never wanes and must be treated for the duration of opioid therapy. Patients on chronic opioids should have scheduled bowel stimulants with agents such as senna, bisacodyl, polyethylene glycol, and/or sorbitol and titrated and escalated as needed.

Opioid Dosing in Patients Who Are Opioid Naive

Patients who are opioid naive may be given 5–10 mg IV depending on the level of their pain with all of the same considerations for pharmacokinetics, initial and subsequent doses.

Equianalgesic Calculations

The ability to perform equianalgesic calculations that allow for adequate breakthrough dosing of opioid medications in the acute setting is fundamental. An equianalgesic dose is the dose at which two opioids at steady state will provide approximately the same pain relief. Equianalgesic dosing tables have been derived to assist clinicians in evaluating all the opioids the patient is on and creating "like units" for a summative amount of medication the patient is using. The stem "equi" for "equal" or "the same" can be misleading, as equianalgesic dosing tables are not exact and should be used as an approximate guide (Table 7.1). When using an equianalgesic dosing table, all opioids are converted to one opioid, morphine, for the purposes of calculations. This conversion of all opioids to morphine is commonly referred to as OMEs or morphine equivalent dose (MED). While more than one equianalgesic dosing table exists, use of one chosen table is recommended consistently across their patients so that physicians become familiar first hand with the dosing and response of a particular table.

Breakthrough Dosing

When all opioids are converted, a breakthrough dose can be calculated (Box 7.1). A breakthrough dose should be considered a "rescue" dose for

TABLE 7.1 **Equianalgesic Dosing Table**

Oral	Drug	IV
30	Morphine	10
20	Oxycodone	—
7.5	Hydromorphone	1.5
30	Hydrocodone	—
Fentanyl 25 µg/hr ~ 50 mg of oral morphine/day		

Source: American Pain Society; 2003.

10-Step Protocol for Opioid Management of Cancer Breakthrough Pain

1. Confirm previous 24-hour use of all opioids.
2. Convert all opioids to oral morphine equivalents (OMEs) used in the previous 24-hour period for the total daily dose (TDD).
3. Calculate breakthrough dose of 5%–20% of the TDD (5% for elderly or renal impairment; 10% typical; 20% for severe pain or patient in severe distress).
4. Reduce by 30%–50% for cross tolerance.
5. Adjust further if needed for renal or hepatic failure.
6. Order/administer the dose.
7. Reassess pain at Tmax—15 minutes IV; 30 minutes SC/IM; 60 minutes oral.
8. At Tmax—pain unchanged or increased → increase the dose by 50%–100%; pain decreased but inadequately controlled→ give same dose; pain improved and adequately controlled → no further dose needed.
9. Continue to reassess for additional doses during patient's emergency department stay.
10. Disposition: consult with patient, oncologist, and/or palliative care based on response to therapy.

pain not controlled on a stable regimen. This breakthrough dose is calculated as a percentage of the total daily dose (TDD)—the total amount of OMEs or MEDs used in a 24-hour period. The breakthrough dose should be taken as a percentage of the TDD between 5%–20%; 5% for elderly or renal impairment; 10% typical; 20% for severe pain or patient in severe distress. Once the breakthrough dose has been determined, if the patient has not taken that particular opioid currently (different opioid) or there is a variation in route (same opioid, different route), the dose should be reduced by 30%–50% for cross tolerance. Emergency clinicians are less likely to provide adequate doses of an initial breakthrough dose at higher OMEs. In one study by Patel et al. patients with daily home use less than 200 OMEs generally received adequate initial breakthrough opioid doses in an ED visit, but patients with higher OMEs were at increased likelihood of being undertreated. Of patients taking <200 OMEs per day, 77.4% received an adequate initial dose but only 3.2% of patients taking >400 OMEs per day prior to the visit received an adequate breakthrough dose. Patients with

>400 OMEs had 99% lower odds of receiving an adequate initial dose of breakthrough opioid in the ED compared to patients with a home OME dose <100 OMEs.

Pharmacokinetic Considerations

Key pharmacokinetic considerations include (1) the time to maximal concentration (Tmax) and (2) opioid clearance. The Tmax is the time to which a single dose reaches its maximal concentration. With opioid dosing of an immediate-release opioid, the plasma concentration of the opioid correlates to analgesia as well as toxicity. For common immediate-release opioids such as hydrocodone, morphine, hydrocodone, and hydromorphone, the Tmax for IV is 5–15 minutes and for oral 30–60 minutes; for IV Fentanyl, the Tmax is 5 minutes. Opioids may be redosed at the Tmax; because if there is no significant effect at the peak time to effect, analgesic is unlikely to be achieved. Clearance concerns can be significant for patients with renal or hepatic failure for any reason. Opioid dosing should be adjusted in renal failure based on the creatinine clearance with a dose reduction. Due to the prevalence and characteristics of active metabolites—oxycodone is not recommended in end-stage renal disease, and fentanyl though short acting is preferred due to its lack of active metabolites (Table 7.2). In the setting of hepatic failure, there are alterations in absorption, distribution, metabolism, and excretion (when severe liver disease leads to renal failure). With hepatic failure the dose should be reduced and the interval between doses lengthened. One helpful guide is "half the dose and twice the interval" for severe hepatic impairment.

TABLE 7.2 **Opioid Dose Adjustment in Renal Failure—Percent of Normal Dose**

GFR (ml/min)	Morphine	Hydrocodone/ Hydromorphone	Oxycodone	Fentanyl
>50	Normal dose	50%–100%	100%	100%
10–50	50%–75%	50%	50%	75%–50%
<10	Not recommended	25% normal dose	Do not use	50%

Initial and Subsequent Doses

The National Cancer Consensus Guidelines for pain management in a patient with a pain crisis recommends that if after an initial dose, pain is unchanged or increased that the breakthrough dose should be increased by 50%–100%; if the pain is decreased but inadequately controlled, the dose should be repeated; and if the pain is improved and adequately controlled, the patient should receive additional doses as needed.

Consultations

When the emergency clinician is uncomfortable or in need of additional guidance, the clinician should consider calling the palliative care consultation service, anesthesia/pain service, and/or the oncologist for guidance. The additional expertise and support of these providers may assist in opioid management, further assessment, and intervention by the interdisciplinary team to support the pain management plan.

CASE CONCLUSION

The clinician verifies that the patient has in fact taken 100 mg of morphine orally every 12 hours and 20 mg of oxycodone every 4 hours around the clock for a total of 200 mg of morphine and 160 mg of oxycodone in a 24-hour period. The patient's serum creatinine is 0.9. The patient reports his pain level is 10/10.

- The conversion of oxycodone 160 mg is 240 mg OMEs for a total of 360 mg OME in 24 hours.
- For the breakthrough dose the clinician uses an average 10% dose of the 24-hour OME = 36 mg of oxycodone with conversion to IV hydromorphone.
- Conversion of oxycodone to hydromorphone: 20 mg oxycodone = 1.5 mg hydromorphone; 36 mg oxycodone = 2.7 mg IV hydromorphone.
- Reduce by 50% for cross tolerance = 1.35 mg.
- Administer dose of 1.5 mg IV for rounding based on the medication denomination available.

Fifteen minutes after the dose is administered, the patient is reassessed, and his pain is now 5/10 and improved, but he is still uncomfortable. Based on this, another dose of 1.5 mg IV is given, and the patient's pain is a 2/10. The ED chaplain visits and supports the patient by attempting a guided meditation to assist with coping with the pain. After 45 minutes the patient's pain returns to 10/10, and he is given an additional dose of 3.0 mg, and a decision to admit is made due to the patient's persistent, severe pain.

KEY POINTS

- Pain may be classified as nociceptive (visceral or somatic), neuropathic, or mixed type.
- Patients who are opioid tolerant and taking >60 OMEs per day are less likely to experience toxicity with appropriate dosing.
- Breakthrough cancer pain can be treated by using an initial dose of 5%–20% (average 10%) of the total OMEs from the previous 24 hours.
- Dose reduction/adjustment may be necessary due to renal or hepatic dysfunction.
- Opioid-induced constipation requires prophylaxis with stimulant-type agents.

Further Reading
1. Burnod A, Maindet C, George B, Minello C, Allano G, Lemaire A. A clinical approach to the management of cancer-related pain in emergency situations. *Support Care Cancer.* 2019;27(8):3147–3157.
2. Coyne CJ, Reyes-Gibby CC, Durham DD, et al. Cancer pain management in the emergency department: A multicenter prospective observational trial of the Comprehensive Oncologic Emergencies Research Network (CONCERN). *Support Care Cancer.* 2021;29(8):4543–4553.
3. Fortner BV, Okon TA, Portenoy RK. A survey of pain-related hospitalizations, emergency department visits, and physician office visits reported by cancer patients with and without history of breakthrough pain. *J Pain.* 2002;3(1):38–44.
4. Patel PM, Goodman LF, Knepel SA, et al. Evaluation of emergency department management of opioid-tolerant cancer patients with acute pain. *J Pain Symptom Manage.* 2017;54(4):501–507.

5. Johnson SJ. Opioid safety in patients with renal or hepatic dysfunction. Pain Treatment Topics. June 2007. http://paincommunity.org/blog/wp-content/uploads/Opioids-Renal-Hepatic-Dysfunction.pdf

6. National Comprehensive Cancer Network. Management of a Cancer Pain Crisis PAIN-5. National Comprehensive Cancer Pain Network Version 1. 2020.

7. Delco F, Tchambaz L, Schlienger R, et al. Dose adjustment in patients with liver disease. *Drug Safety*. 2005;28(6):529–545.

8. Vardy J, Agar M. Nonopioid drugs in the treatment of cancer pain. *J Clin Oncol*. 2014;32(16):1677–1690.

9. Camilleri M. Opioid-induced constipation: Challenges and therapeutic opportunities. *Am J Gastroenterol*. 2011;106(5):835–842.

10. Burnod A, Maindet C, George B, Minello C, Allano G, Lemaire A. A clinical approach to the management of cancer-related pain in emergency situations. *Support Care Cancer*. 2019;27(8):3147–3157.

8 When Time Is Short

Monique Schaulis

Case: A 63-year-old man with metastatic colon cancer presents to the emergency department (ED) with rapid respirations and moaning. His wife reports that he has been at home and worsening for the last 2 weeks. A home care nurse and physician have been managing his symptoms of shortness of breath and pain. The patient and his wife were told 1 month ago that there were no more options for cancer-directed therapy and that the focus of care would be on his symptoms. Over the last day, he has stopped eating and drinking and has been increasingly agitated and confused. In the ED his blood pressure is 60/40 mmHg, heart rate is 135 beats per minute, respiratory rate is 35 per minute, and oxygen saturation is 90% on 2L. He is moaning and thrashing about in the bed. He has paradoxical abdominal breathing with accessory muscle use and looks fearful. He has noisy upper airway secretions. His wife reports that she feels he is dying and wants him to be comfortable, but she does not feel she can care for him at home.

What do you do now?

LAST HOURS OF LIVING

Over 50% of older adults are seen in the ED in the last month of life, and more than 75% in the last 6 months. The constellation of signs and symptoms of dyspnea, delirium, decreasing oral intake, and changes in vital signs in malignant and nonmalignant illnesses signifies impending death, most likely in hours to days. Rapid assessment of prognosis and goals-of-care guides the next steps. While dying is the expected outcome of his advanced and untreatable cancer, how dying will be managed depends upon patient and surrogate factors. If the goal is comfort, urgent symptom management takes priority over resuscitative measures, and decreasing suffering becomes the focus. The ED team pivots from resuscitation to palliation. Interventions such as diagnostic workup may be modified or aborted as they may cause more distress. Key steps include (1) recognition of active dying, (2) concurrent aggressive symptom assessment, (3) management with rapid high-quality goals-of-care conversation, and (4) preparation for an ED death or outside disposition.

RECOGNITION OF ACTIVE DYING

There are many physiologic changes associated with active dying that the emergency physician should recognize. Patients are weak and usually unable to lift their head off the bed. Urine output will be low or absent. Tachycardia and hypotension are common. Respirations may become irregular, and rapid breaths may be followed by periods of apnea. Swallowing is impaired and patients may have loud rattling breathing from pooled secretions in the hypopharynx. Skin often becomes mottled and discolored. Neurologic changes typically manifest as one of two patterns that have been described as the "two roads to death" (Figure 8.1). Of dying patients, 70%–90% follow the "usual road" and die quietly, and 10%–30% follow the "difficult road" and become terminally delirious.

When on the "difficult" road, patients experience agitated delirium that may progress from confusion to hallucinations, tremors, myoclonic jerks, and even seizures prior to death. In this case, the patient is moaning and thrashing, suggesting agitated delirium.

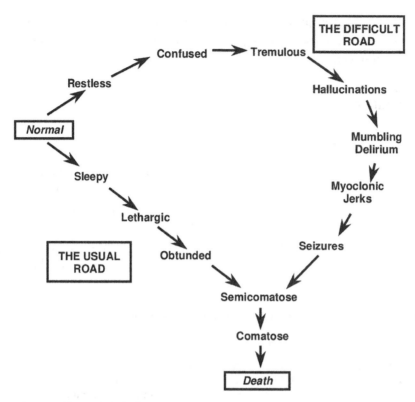

FIGURE 8.1. Two roads to death.

Labored breathing is another common sign of being close to death. Labored breathing may be, but is not always, a sign of dyspnea. Dyspnea is a subjective symptom distinct from respiratory rate. Assessment of dyspnea and respiratory distress can be challenging as patients usually lose the ability to report shortness of breath but not the ability to experience it. The Respiratory Distress Observation Scale (RDOS) is a tool, validated for end of life, that guides symptom management and assessment of comfort.

Pain can be assessed using both verbal and nonverbal scales. Care should be taken to distinguish pain from delirium or respiratory distress. When pain is present opioids, may be titrated quickly until symptoms improve. In this case, morphine is a first-line medication. Keep in mind that the patient is dying; one cannot expect or aim for normalization of vital signs. A clear decision to give opioids despite hypotension should be made and communicated to the nurse so vital sign parameters do not interfere with symptom management.

AGGRESSIVE SYMPTOM TREATMENT

See Table 8.1.[2]

Common symptoms at the end of life include neurological changes (lethargy/delirium), dyspnea, terminal secretions, and pain. Given the severity of the symptoms that may be present as well as the routine use of the IV route in the ED, IV medication is preferred for rapid onset and close titration (Table 8.2). If IV access is challenging or invasive, subcutaneous infusion can be used, or medicines may be given rectally. Oral routes can also be used, but keep in mind that the time of onset can be up to 1 hour.

TABLE 8.1 **Medications Used during the Last Hours of Life**

Drug	Dosing	Notes
Lorazepam	1–2 mg buccal mucosal, PR, SL, SC, IV, q1 h to titrate, then q4–6h to maintain	If paradoxical agitation observed, choose a nonbenzodiazepine for sedation
Haloperidol	2–5 mg PR, SC, IV qlh to titrate, then q6h to maintain	Relatively nonsedating at low doses. May require 10–30 mg daily to sedate
Chlorpromazine	10–25 mg PR, IV q4–6h	Parenteral route may require special exemptions from standard nursing policy in some settings
Scopolamine (hyoscine hydrobromide)	10–100 p.g/h SC, IV continuous infusion or 0.1–0.4 mg SC q6h or 1–10 patches q72h	Transdermal preparation only delivers approximately 10 p,g/h and takes many hours to reach therapeutic levels
Glycopyrrolate	0.2–0.4 mg SC q2–4h and titrate	Does not cross blood-brain barrier

Abbreviations: IV, intravenous; PR, per rectum; SC, subcutaneous; SL, sublingual.

TABLE 8.2 **Pharmacologic Agents for Noisy Secretions**

Drug	Trade Name	Route	Starting Dose	Onset
Scopolamine (hyoscine) Hydrobromide	Transderm Scop	Patch	One 1.5 mg patch	–12 h (24 h to steady state)
Hyoscyamine	Levsin	PO, SL	0.125 mg	30 min
Glycopyrrolate	Robinul	PO	1 mg	30 min
Glycopyrrolate	Robinul	SubQ, IV	0.2 mg	1 min
Atropine sulfate	Atropine	SubQ, IV	0.1 mg	1 min
Atropine sulfate	multiple	Sublingual	1 gtt (1% ophth. solution)	30 min

DELIRIUM

In this case, our patient is experiencing agitated delirium. Haldol and benzodiazepines are effective for sedation if needed for agitated delirium. Neuroleptics are preferred over benzodiazepines due to the potential for paradoxical effects. In cases of severe agitation refractory to neuroleptics, or when neuroleptics are clearly contraindicated, benzodiazepines should be used. Haldol dose can begin at 1 mg IV or SC if there is no IV access. Ativan can be given IV or subcutaneously starting at 0.5–1 mg.[3]

SECRETION MANAGEMENT

Noisy respiratory or pharyngeal secretions are common during the last days of life and are commonly known as the death rattle. Establish whether the noise is distressing the dying person or his caregivers. It is important to reassure families that though the noise may be disturbing, it is unlikely to cause discomfort. Be prepared to listen to their concerns and fears. Repositioning on the side may be helpful. Deep suctioning is not recommended as it can cause discomfort. Pharmacologic treatment for secretions may be useful but does not have strong evidence. Glycopyrrolate is the preferred agent because it does not cross the blood-brain barrier, but atropine ophthalmic drops are also commonly used for convenience. When using pharmacological agents for noisy secretions, monitor for improvements and discontinue if the treatment is not working (Table 8.3). Treat side effects like delirium, agitation, sedation, or dry mouth if they occur.[4]

DYSPNEA

Opioids are the drugs of choice for dyspnea at the end of life. In the opioid-naïve patient, low doses of oral (5–10 mg) or parenteral morphine (2–4 mg) will provide relief for most patients; higher doses will be needed for patients on chronic opioids. When dyspnea is acute and severe, parenteral is the route of choice: 1–2 mg IV every 15 minutes if needed until relief in the opioid-naïve patient. In opioid-tolerant patients, administration of 5% of the total daily morphine equivalents IV can be given per dose. Sensitive communication regarding the burdens and benefits of oxygen should be assessed. Oxygen is often, but not universally, helpful for dyspnea but can remain a symbol of care that families may perceive to be "doing something." A therapeutic trial, based on symptom relief, not pulse oximetry, is indicated in dying patients. However, if agitation is present, the nasal cannula may exacerbate it.[1]

PAIN

Pain can be assessed using both verbal and nonverbal scales. Care should be taken to distinguish pain from delirium or respiratory distress. To differentiate the moaning and groaning of terminal delirium from pain, it is helpful to look for tension across the forehead, furrowing of the eyebrows, or facial grimacing. If these signs are absent, the vocalization is more likely to be related to delirium than pain.[1]

When pain is present, opioids may be titrated quickly until symptoms improve. As you treat symptoms, keep in mind that the patient is dying; you cannot expect or aim for normalization of vital signs. A clear decision to give opioids despite hypotension should be conveyed to the nurse so that vital sign parameters do not interfere with symptom management. A clinician may be tempted to give IV fluids for hypotension, but this may make symptoms worse, particularly dyspnea, and may prolong the dying process.

COMMUNICATION

Communication during active dying can be both one of the most challenging and rewarding aspects of work in the ED and merits its own chapter. In the setting of active dying, the clinician cannot defer this conversation to later in the hospital course. The clinician must both simultaneously treat distressing symptoms and assess goals of care. A rapid, structured conversation may seem overwhelming but in practice usually takes less than 10 minutes. Having a communication map will help the emergency physician conduct this important conversation faster than it takes to place a central line or repair many lacerations. As with any procedure, these conversations can seem awkward at first, but with practice, they become easier and more natural. A recommended communication framework for a rapid goals-of-care conversation is REMAP, covered in Chapter 3.

DISPOSITION/PREPARATION FOR AN EMERGENCY DEPARTMENT DEATH

Disposition will be affected by prognosis, symptom control, and family dynamics, as well as by your local practice environment and community resources. In this case, given his severe symptoms, hemodynamic instability, and goals, strong consideration should be given to a recommendation for admission to a palliative unit or to the regular inpatient service for comfort-focused care. Support by an ED social work and/or case management will be critical and consultation of a palliative care service if available. If the foremost goal is a home death, consideration should be given to urgent home hospice intake. If this is the case, transporting the patient while acknowledging the risk of death en route may be considered. If transport is considered, good communication with the family and EMS regarding goals and expectations is critical, and in some states, documents like a POLST will be important.

Often, time is short, beds are few, and death in the ED will inevitably happen. Dying in the chaotic ED environment can have a lasting effect on patients and families. Alarming, beeping, screaming, moaning, and seemingly inappropriate chatting and laughing can be distressing to all patients and families. Planning around noise control for dying patients and families should be an institutional goal as well as one that staff prioritize in

BOX 8.1   **RESPECT Project: An Approach to Death in the Emergency Department**

R: Restore order: Prepare loved ones for coming to the bedside.
E: Explain: What happened and who was involved in patient's care.
S: Stop and set aside other duties: Other things can wait.
P: Be present: Give your full awareness to what's unfolding before you.
E: Empathize: Take a moment to acknowledge that a life has just ended.
C: Chaplain/clergy: Offer to call for spiritual support.
T: Time: Allow family time with their loved one before moving on to other business.

Source: Schmidt S. The Respect Project. Kaiser San Rafael Emergency Department. 2016. http://www.sfmms.org/Portals/27/assets/mms/magazine/magazine-images/RESP ECT%20Protocol.pdf?ver=2016-06-27-124837-067.

the moment. An ED that recognizes the importance of providing comfort during dying as part of a mandate for excellent care decreases the burden on individual providers and standardizes our ED response. Rather than treating ED death as a failure, or as a situation where there is "nothing more we can do," the ED interdisciplinary team, including physicians, nurses, techs, environmental services, and social services can work together to actively support patients and families. Culture and systems change can help families and staff begin to heal by decreasing the trauma they experience in the ED. Box 8.1 shows an example of a quality improvement project focused on death in the ED.

CASE DISCUSSION

In this vignette, the patient arrives at the ED unstable and in distress. You quickly address his dyspnea using the RDOS scale with an initial RDOS score of 12 and administer morphine 2 mg IV q 15 minutes for two doses where his RDOS score comes to 2. He has persistent agitation. You administer one dose of haloperidol of 0.5 mg IV. For his noisy respirations you administer one dose of glycopyrrolate 0.2 mg IV that reduces the secretions, though they are still present.

As you aggressively manage his symptoms, you concurrently have a goals-of-care conversation with his wife. You start the conversation with his wife by *asking permission* to discuss what's happening: "Would it be okay if we spent a few minutes talking about your husband's condition?" This signals that the conversation is important and, at the same time, gives the wife a sense of control. The next step is to *assess his wife's understanding of the illness.* You might ask, "What have you heard about his illness and what to expect?" In this case, his wife reports that she understands there is no more cancer-directed treatment and that the focus of care is on his symptoms. Because his wife says directly that she feels he is dying, you see that she already understands the terminal illness. To confirm that you are both on the same page, you might agree by *giving a clear headline* like "Yes, you're right. He is in the process of dying and does not have much time left." After giving the headline, it is helpful to *remain silent* to let the information sink in. You prepare to *respond to the wife's emotion using empathy.* The NURSE tool provides a variety of types of phrases to help the emergency physician respond with explicit empathy in emotional situations. "It must be so hard to see him like this." You address the wife to *find out what is most important* by asking something like "Knowing that time is short, what would he say is most important now?" She has expressed that keeping her husband comfortable as he dies is most important. This is a good time to inquire about spiritual concerns and to offer chaplaincy as available. Another question in this setting may be, "Is it important to him where he dies?" This will help guide your options for disposition. Next, use an *aligning statement* to show the wife that you have heard what is most important. In this case, you might say, "It sounds like what is most important right now is getting his symptoms under control so that he can die comfortably and you don't feel like home is best now—do I have that right?" This helps the wife feel heard and will let her know that you are basing your recommendation on what she has told you. Based on this information, *make a recommendation* for next steps. As you work together to make a plan, explain to her *what you will do* as part of keeping him comfortable: aggressive symptom management with medications and oxygen, admit to a palliative unit for end-of-life care *before you tell her what you won't do* or recommend to include no transfer to the intensive care unit, resuscitation, or other life-extending therapies. This all leads to a plan to allow natural death and focus on comfort. You educate his wife on the signed of normal dying, the significance that secretions do not mean he is suffering and reassure her that you will continue to ensure his comfort.

There are no beds available in the hospital, inpatient community hospice, or palliative care unit. The RESPECT protocol is initiated. A placard is placed on his door to remind staff of what to do and what not to do. Monitors and beeping are turned off, and noise control is initiated. Regular blood pressure monitoring stops. Lactates are not trended, and IV fluids are not ordered. A tech offers seating to any family or friends. Social work is available, and spiritual support is offered. Water, food, and wifi/phone are made available to the family. The nurse monitors symptoms closely, recognizes nonverbal signs of pain, such as shortness of breath with key aspects of assessment being furrowing of brow, grimacing, calling out, tensing of muscles, or agitation, and notifies the physician. After an hour, the patient dies peacefully.

After his death, his wife stays with him for the time she needs. Social work is easily available to help with arrangements. Staff takes a moment to debrief and recognize the moment as well as the work they have done for both the patient and his wife. The patient's wife will grieve, but she will not suffer from guilt about trauma he endured in the ED as he was dying.

KEY POINTS

- Aggressive physical symptom control is often needed at end of life to include pain, shortness of breath, agitation/delirium and secretion management.
- Families and caregivers of actively dying patients are best supported by an empathic conversation focused on goals, priorities with clear recommendations by the ED provider.
- Control environment: noise, privacy, temperature, and seating.
- Encourage a culture of teamwork around death and dying in the ED.
- Protocols focused on the comfort of dying patients and their loved ones (or those who have died) are recommended to standardize ED approach.

Further Reading

1. Smith AK et al. Half of older Americans seen in emergency department in last month of life; most admitted to hospital, and many die there. *Health Affairs (Project Hope)*. 2012;31(6):1277–1285. doi:10.1377/hlthaff.2011.0922.

2. Ferris FD. Last hours of living. *Clin Geriatr Med*. 2004 Nov;20(4):641–667, vi. doi:10.1016/j.cger.2004.07.011. PMID: 15541617. https://www.mypcnow.org/fast-fact/physical-examination-of-the-dying-patient/

3. Hui D et al. Effect of lorazepam with haloperidol vs haloperidol alone on agitated delirium in patients with advanced cancer receiving palliative care: A randomized clinical trial. *JAMA*. 2017;318(11):1047–1056.

4. National Clinical Guideline Centre. *Care of Dying Adults in the Last Days of Life*. National Institute for Health and Care Excellence: UK; 2015 Dec 16. (NICE Guideline, No. 31.) 9, Pharmacological interventions. https://www.ncbi.nlm.nih.gov/books/NBK355997/

5. Grudzen CR, Emlet LL, Kuntz J, et al. EM talk: Communication skills training for emergency medicine patients with serious illness. *BMJ Support Palliat Care*. 2016;6(2):219–224. doi:10.1136/bmjspcare-2015-000993

6. Campbell ML, Templin T, Walch J. *Journal of Palliative Medicine*. 2010;13(3):285–290. http://doi.org/10.1089/jpm.2009.0229

7. Lamba S, Quest TE. Hospice care and the emergency department: Rules, regulations, and referrals. *Ann Emerg Med*. 2011;57(3):282–290. doi:10.1016/j.annemergmed.2010.06.569. PMID: 21035900.

8. Mierendorf SM, Gidvani V. Palliative care in the emergency department. *The Permanente Journal*. 2014;18(2):77–85. doi:10.7812/TPP/13-103.

9 "I Don't Like It Hot"

Gretchen E. Bell and Paul L. DeSandre

Case: A 59-year-old woman with a history of primary, progressive multiple sclerosis presents to the emergency department (ED) with reports of uncontrolled pain in her legs that is burning, stabbing, and sharp in nature and is not relieved by any home interventions. Her caregiver accompanies her and reports that she is bedbound and cries mostly every night in pain. She has been giving increasing doses of morphine 15 mg immediate release every 4 hours. For the last 2 days, she has been administering the morphine every 2 hours around the clock. Despite this, the pain seems to be worsening. She has also been taking gabapentin 600 mg every 8 hours for the last 6 weeks with no relief.

What do you do now?

NONMALIGNANT CHRONIC PAIN IN THE SERIOUSLY ILL

This patient's pain is uncontrolled and related to her primary progressive multiple sclerosis. Pain is among the most common reasons for seeking emergency care and is prevalent in the palliative care population. Pain is defined by the International Association for the Study of Pain (IASP) as "an unpleasant sensory and emotional experience associated with actual or potential tissue damage, and described in terms of such damage, or both." While variations exist in the definition of chronic pain, the Centers for Disease Control and Prevention (CDC) defines it as lasting greater than 3 months. Therefore, in this case, the pain may be classified as nonmalignant chronic pain. Like many chronic conditions, chronic pain management is best managed comprehensively with a multimodal approach by a consistent outpatient provider. However, when pain symptoms become unmanageable, the ED becomes a readily accessible resource for seeking relief.

Acute pain involves activation of nociceptors and the autonomic nervous system and is at least partially adaptive. The pathophysiology of chronic pain is more complex, involving pathologic changes in pain receptors and the central and peripheral nervous system that may or may not be related to distinct tissue pathology or injury. In addition to acute or chronic, pain may be classified as nociceptive or neuropathic. These distinctions are important in determining the appropriate management strategies. Nociceptive pain is primarily an acute pain experience that is in response to the threat of or actual tissue damage. Nociceptive pain may be somatic or visceral. If somatic, it may be described as sharp, aching, or throbbing, and localized. The receptors are primarily in bone, muscle, soft tissue, and skin. If visceral, it may be more aching and vaguely localizable. Neuropathic pain, by contrast, is more typically described as burning, tingling, or shooting. Neuropathic pain may be acute, such as with direct nerve damage, or chronic dysfunction. When chronic, it is characterized by alterations in how stimuli is perceived and responded, and it is associated with changes of the central and peripheral nervous system. Understanding certain neuropathic pain syndromes may help in interpreting a patient's pain description.

Hyperalgesia is an exaggerated response to stimulation. Opioid-induced hyperalgesia is a paradoxical escalation of pain with increasing opioid dosing. Proposed mechanisms include the accumulation of neurotoxic opioid metabolites and activation of N-methyl-D-aspartate (NMDA) receptors in the central nervous system. Allodynia is a painful response to typically nonpainful stimulus, like light touch or moderate temperature changes. Causalgia (or complex regional pain syndrome) is pain in the absence of stimuli due to spontaneous nerve firing. Patients can experience more than one type of pain simultaneously. In the example of multiple sclerosis, the patient may have neuropathic pain as a result of direct nerve dysfunction; somatic pain due to myofascial scarring and immobility, tissue pressure, and muscle spasm; chronic pain syndromes related to altered responses and feedback loops in central and peripheral nervous systems due to chronic stimulation; and possibly opioid-induced hyperalgesia.

Eliciting a chronic pain history in the ED may feel daunting, but with appropriate focus and collaboration, the care of the patient can be both efficient and effective. As with other patients presenting to the ED, the first step in the assessment of chronic pain is to determine the reason for seeking emergency care. The initial priority is to determine if the cause of the pain is known or new. If known, is the pain inadequately or incorrectly managed (by either the patient or the prescriber)? Is the patient addressing pain symptoms with aberrant coping strategies and misusing medications? Is this an escalation of previously controlled pain of a known etiology? If new, is this a life or limb threat requiring emergent investigation, or is this a less urgent concern best addressed in outpatient follow-up? In addition, speaking with the primary care provider (PCP) can provide valuable additional history and assist in implementing a consistent treatment plan.

When considering treatment strategies, pain intensity scales may be less useful in chronic nonmalignant pain than with acute pain. Functional changes in activities of daily living are generally a better gauge of the efficacy of treatment. In addition, pain intensity may be affected by physical, psychological, social, and even spiritual distress. Chronic pain can create a vicious cycle affecting all of these domains over time. It is important for the ED provider to respect the influence of chronic pain on more general suffering and to support a multimodal approach to treatment and consistent outpatient follow-up.

Chronic pain is optimally managed outpatient with an interdisciplinary care team supervised by a PCP, including physical or occupation therapy, behavioral therapy, social work, nutrition, spiritual health providers, and pharmacy. In the ED, seek to identify unmet needs and ensure involvement of adequate resources to optimize care, including referral for substance use disorder when appropriate.

Medical management should include consideration of nonopioid analgesics and adjuvant agents tailored to the patient's specific type of pain and comorbidities. Neuropathic pain may respond better to adjuvant agents than opiates. Table 9.1 provides information on specific medications, side effect profile, and dosing strategies.

Opioids are generally less helpful in reducing the intensity of chronic pain, but they may be useful in improving overall function. When effective, opioids may be part of a multimodal treatment plan. Opioids should not be started for chronic pain without consulting the patient's PCP. Based on a careful clinical assessment and review of the local Prescription Drug Monitoring Program data, if refilling an existing opioid prescription is supportable, the quantity should be limited to allow follow-up at the next available business day with the PCP.

The patient in the vignette has poorly controlled chronic pain with significant impact on her mobility and sleep. She is using gabapentin 600 mg every 8 hours without evident adverse response, and she has taken 12 doses of 15 mg morphine tablets (180 mg) in escalating frequency during the last 24 hours with worsening pain. If the patient were previously opioid responsive, the description of worsening pain would support opioid hyperalgesia syndrome. An effective intervention strategy in opioid hyperalgesia is to choose an alternate opioid at 50% reduction in daily dose. For immediate intervention, a breakthrough dose of an alternate opioid (which is typically 10% of the daily requirement) may be given, such as hydromorphone 1 mg IV (10% of 180 mg oral morphine/24 hours = 18 mg oral morphine = 0.9 mg IV hydromorphone). Renal and hepatic function should be assessed before determining an outpatient plan with the PCP. In this scenario, a reasonable consideration may be oxycodone extended release 30 mg every 12 hours (50% of 180 mg oral morphine/24 hours = 90 mg oral morphine = 60 mg oral oxycodone). For breakthrough pain (usually 10% of daily requirement), oxycodone 5 mg every 4 hours as needed for severe pain or >7/10 (10% of 60 mg oxycodone extended release = 6 mg oxycodone immediate release). Adequate dispense in the prescription should allow the patient to present to the PCP office the next business day. Maximal

TABLE 9.1 Overview of first Line Adjuvant Agents for Treating Neuropathic Pain

Class/Medication		Mechanism of Action	Dosing Strategy				Caution/Effects
			Initial	Titration	Goal*	Trial	
TCA's	Nortriptyline	Increase CNS synaptic of serotonin and/or norepinephrine.	25 mg daily	25 mg q 3–7 days	150 mg/day	6–8 weeks; 2 at max tolerated dose	Caution: Cardiac disease, glaucoma, suicide risk, seizure disorder, geriatric[H] Adverse Effects: Sedation, dry mouth, blurred vision, weight gain, urinary retention;
	Desipramine		12.5 mg QHS	25 mg q 2-7 days	150 mg/day		
	Amitriptyline	Decrease acetylcholine 5-hydroxytryptamine and histamine,	10–25 mg QHS	25 mg q7 days	150 mg/day		
SNRI's	Duloxetine	Increase levels of serotonin and norepinephrine by preventing uptake, weak inhibitors of dopamine reuptake	30 mg daily	30 mg after 7 days	60 mg /day	4 weeks	Caution: Hepatic dysfunction, renal insufficiency, alcohol abuse; Adverse Effect; Nausea
	Venlafaxine		37.5 mg daily	75 mg q7 days	225 mg daily	4–6 weeks	Caution: Cardiac disease;

(continued)

TABLE 9.1 Continued

Class/Medication		Mechanism of Action	Dosing Strategy				Caution/Effects
			Initial	Titration	Goal*	Trial	
Calcium channel a2-d ligands	Gabapentin	Believed to bind at the alpha-2-delta subunit of voltage-gated calcium channels inhibiting excitatory neurotransmitter release	100–300 mg QHS	100 mg TID q1–2	3600 mg/day	4–8 weeks; 2 at max tolerated dose	Caution: Myasthenia Gravis. Substance abuse hx, CKD1[I] Adverse Effects:
	Pregabalin		75 mg BID	150 mg q3– 7 days	600 mg/day	4 weeks	Sedation, dizziness, peripheral edema; angioedema**

Abbreviations: TCA, Tricyclic Antidepressant; SNRIs, Serotonin-Noreprinephrine reuptake Inhibitors.

*Goal dosing is listed as the total daily recommended dose and dose include recommended dosing interval.

[H]Due to increasesd risk of side effects, consider decreasing the starting dose and giving in divided dose in geriatric patients.

[I]Dose should be adjusted by creatinine clearance.

**Has been reported with both initial and chronic therapy. Use with caution in patiens with a history of angioedema.

Prepared with data from:

Dworking RH, O'Connor AG, Backonja M. et al. Pharmacologic management of neuropathic pain: Evidence-based recommendations. Pain. 2007;132(3): 237–251.

DynaMed [database online]. Ipswich (MA); EBSCO Information Services. http://www.dynamed.com. Accessed December 14, 2019.

Lexicomp Online. Copyright © 1978–2019 Leicomp, Inc. All Rights Reserved.

dosing of gabapentin is approximately 3600 mg/day. Therefore, a reasonable gabapentin dose increase in this case would be from 600 mg to 900 mg every 8 hours. Unless other reasons emerge to admit the patient, most chronic pain patients should be able to be discharged to home from the ED and referred to their PCP for follow-up.

KEY POINTS

- Chronic nonmalignant pain complaints require a detailed pain history that includes screening for usual life or limb threats.
- Unlike acute pain, assessment should focus more on functional changes and less on pain intensity.
- Improvement is a long-term goal, and it requires comprehensive management and coordination with a PCP.
- Some patients with chronic pain may be opioid responsive with improved function on appropriate doses.
- Adjuvant pharmacological and nonpharmacological therapies play an important role in the management of chronic pain.

Further Reading

1. Clauw DJ, Essex MN, Pitman V, Jones KD. Reframing chronic pain as a disease, not a symptom: Rationale and implications for pain management. *Postgrad Med.* 2019;131(3):185–198. doi:10.1080/00325481.2019.1574403.
2. Dépelteau A, Racine-Hemmings F, Lagueux É, Hudon C. Chronic pain and frequent use of emergency department: A systematic review. *Am J Emerg Med.* 2019;S0735-6757(19):30641–30642. doi:10.1016/j.ajem.2019.158492.
3. Dworkin RH, O'Connor AB, Backonja M, et al. Pharmacologic management of neuropathic pain: Evidence-based recommendations. *Pain.* 2007;132(3):237–251. doi:10.1016/j.pain.2007.08.033.
4. Hansen GR. Management of chronic pain in the acute care setting. *Emerg Med Clin North Am.* 2005;23(2):307–338. doi:10.1016/j.emc.2004.12.004.
5. McLeod D, Nelson K. The role of the emergency department in the acute management of chronic or recurrent pain. *Australas Emerg Nurs J.* 2013;16(1):30–36. doi:10.1016/j.aenj.2012.12.001.
6. Todd KH. Chronic pain and aberrant drug-related behavior in the emergency department. *J Law Med Ethics.* 2005;33(4):761–769. doi:10.1111/j.1748-720x.2005.tb00542.x.

10 All Stopped Up

Laura Brachman

Case: A 48-year-old woman with metastatic ovarian cancer and chronic bowel obstruction at the level of the duodenum presents to the emergency department (ED) with a 3-day history of increasing shortness of breath and malaise. She reports that she has a persistent left pleural effusion managed by indwelling home pleural drainage system. She drains 500 cc of fluid from the left chest cavity every 3 days. For symptom relief of the obstruction, she has a venting percutaneous gastrostomy tube that continues to drain well. She also elected home total parenteral nutrition via a peripherally inserted central catheter (PICC) line that was started on discharge from the hospital 1 week ago. Her vital signs are temperature of 99.0 °F, blood pressure of 120/75 mmHg, heart rate of 120 beats per minute, and respiratory rate of 14 breaths per minute. She is awake, alert, and in no distress. She reports that her left pleural drain is no longer working. Chest radiography reveals that she has a marked effusion on the left. She is noted to have some redness around the PICC line in the right upper extremity.

What do you do now?

KEY ASPECTS OF PALLIATIVE DEVICES AND THERAPIES IN ADVANCED ILLNESS

Malignant pleural effusions portend a poor prognosis, typically 4–6 months at the time of diagnosis. These effusions have a significant effect on quality of life, with dyspnea and cough being the most common symptoms. When such an effusion is recurrent, an indwelling pleural catheter (IPC) can be placed as an outpatient and drained at home with minimal training. This intervention allows for symptom control without the need for recurrent hospital or office visits. Complications typically occur either at the time of catheter placement (wound infection, bleeding, organ injury, pneumothorax) or after the patient has returned home. The latter are uncommon and include IPC-related pleural infection, loculation, and less commonly catheter tract metastasis. IPC-related pleural infections are typically mild and can be treated with oral antibiotics, although the presence of an empyema can require hospitalization for IV antibiotics and continuous pleural drainage. Symptomatic loculations occur when there is pleural symphysis due to the presence of the IPC. In this case residual pleural fluid is unable to drain through the IPC, leaving the patient short of breath. This is typically seen about 2 months after IPC insertion and has been reported in 5%–14% of IPC-treated patients. Treatment includes with pleural aspiration, removal of the ineffective IPC, and placement of a second catheter. Reported incidence of catheter tract metastases is <5% and typically occurs late (median 280 days) after IPC insertion. The typical presentation is a painful mass near the IPC insertion site. Computed tomography imaging can assist in diagnosis. Treatment is usually with analgesics and external beam radiation without the need to remove the IPC. In deciding how to proceed with these IPC-related complications, it is important to determine if the IPC was alleviating dyspnea or other symptoms attributable to the effusion. If so, then correction of the complication is indicated. However, if, despite drainage, dyspnea persists, functional status has progressively worsened, or the patient is approaching death, it may not make sense to pursue interventions such as hospitalization, radiation therapy, or placement of another IPC. Transition to home-based hospice care may be the best way to achieve the patient's goals of care (GOC), given the changed circumstances.

Table 10.1 presents an overview of devices and therapies used in advanced illness, common complications for which patients present to the emergency room and considerations given to whether GOC have been met. These considerations are important because they will guide next steps in patient management. Triaging these patients involves determining if there is an intervention available in the ED to allow the patient to return home with the device or, if GOC are not being met, considering next steps.

As seen in Table 10.1, other commonly used devices used in advanced illness include indwelling abdominal catheters for recurrent ascites, percutaneous endoscopic gastrostomy (PEG) tubes, jejunal feeding tubes, PICC lines for the administration of total parenteral nutrition (TPN), inotropes and other medications, and percutaneous nephrostomy tubes. The remainder of this chapter will present the approach to complications of some of these other devices in the setting of a patient's GOC.

TOTAL PARENTERAL NUTRITION

Use of TPN at home is unlikely in itself to be a reason for ED presentation. However infection of the catheter through which TPN is administered may well result in an ED visit as catheter-related infections are the most common complication of these devices. If TPN is being received on a permanent basis such as in cases of malabsorption or short bowel syndrome, then appropriate triaging is needed to manage the infection. If there is no evidence of systemic infection and no need for catheter removal, the patient can likely be discharged home from the ED on an appropriate antibiotic regimen. Systemic infections or cases when the catheter must be removed (suspicion of a fungal infection, tunnel tract infection) may require hospital admission. In patients for whom TPN is being provided in the setting of advanced and progressive illness (malignant bowel obstruction), a reconsideration of GOC would be appropriate. For many patients with advanced illness and sepsis from TPN, this could be an endpoint of no longer being able to offer the TPN. This will require a discussion regarding the benefits and burdens of artificial nutrition and hydration in the setting of GOC.

TABLE 10.1   Devices and Therapies Used in Advanced Illness

Device	Purpose	GOC in the Setting of Advanced Illness	Determination of Effectiveness	Potential Complications	Intervention Options
Indwelling pleural drain	Management of recurrent malignant pleural effusion	Outpatient symptom management (dyspnea, cough)	Improved functional status and reduced hospital presentations	Pleural infection, loculation, catheter tract metastases	Oral antibiotics vs. hospitalization for further management
Indwelling abdominal drain	Management of recurrent malignant ascites	Outpatient symptom management (nausea & vomiting, early satiety, dyspnea, pain)	Improved symptoms without recurrent hospital presentations	Infection at tube insertion site, bacterial peritonitis, tube dislodged, obstruction	Antibiotics (oral or IV), tube irrigation, tube replacement
Venting percutaneous gastrostomy tube	Management/ prevention of recurrent bowel obstruction due to advanced cancer	Reduced abdominal pain, nausea and vomiting, administration of medications (including those for symptom management i.e., opioids), allows for comfort feeds	Improved symptom management, prevention of bowel obstruction; fewer hospitalizations	Peristomal leakage, inadequate drainage, tube dislodgement, peritonitis	Bedside flushing and repositioning vs. hospital admission

Feeding tube	Administration of enteral nutrition	Provision of artificial nutrition until ability to swallow is regained, or life prolongation	Treatment of underlying pathology leads to regained swallowing function; patient is more alert in the setting of dementia or delirium	Tube dislodged, clogged tube, peristomal leakage	Tube replacement in ED for mature tract or flushing in ED or need for admission if tract is not mature
PICC line	IV access for medication or parenteral nutrition	Symptom management via IV parenteral medications when oral route not available, life prolongation w/ parenteral nutrition	Adequate symptom management; w/ regard to parenteral nutrition, acceptable quality of life	Systemic infection, PICC line infection, line removed/ dislodged	Antibiotics, tube replacement
Inotropes	Improved cardiac function, reduced symptoms, life prolongation	Relief of volume overload, life prolongation	Less dyspnea, less edema, improved functional status	Loss of central IV access	Temporary use of peripheral IV access
LVAD	Bridge to transplant vs. destination therapy	Bridge to transplant or life prolongation	Less dyspnea, adequate quality of life given restrictions of living w/ LVAD	Drive line infection	Consultation with cardiology; hospitalization most likely required

ABDOMINAL DRAIN

As with refractory malignant pleural effusions, prognosis in the setting of malignant ascites is measured in months, typically 1–4, although it can be longer for ovarian and breast cancer if the patient is receiving systemic therapy. Symptoms associated with malignant ascites include early satiety, nausea and vomiting, dyspnea, and pain. Paracentesis can relieve symptoms and, as with malignant pleural effusions, if ascites is recurrent, an indwelling drainage catheter can be used for symptom palliation while the patient remains at home. The most common complications of indwelling peritoneal catheters include catheter-related infection and obstruction of the catheter such that it does not drain. Infection leading to peritonitis or sepsis in advanced illness requires a GOC conversation regarding the benefits and burdens of hospitalization and treating infection, sepsis, or catheter obstruction. If being at home is preferred over hospitalization and life prolongation, some patients might opt for oral antibiotics or no antibiotics at all along with pain and symptom control. An obstructed catheter sometimes responds to bedside flushing, but in one series about half of patients required catheter removal and replacement, and for some patients this might not be an option.

PERCUTANEOUS ENDOSCOPIC GASTROSTOMY TUBES AND VENTING PERCUTANEOUS ENDOSCOPIC GASTROSTOMY TUBES

PEG tubes are most often used for enteral feeding alone. However, in the palliative care setting a venting PEG is an important management tool in the setting of malignant bowel obstruction (MBO), which occurs in up to 15% of patients with advanced cancer. Initial management of MBO includes conservative measures such as bowel rest, nasogastric tube, and IV fluids. Surgical intervention or stenting may not be feasible in these patients as they usually have a poor performance status. A venting PEG can significantly alleviate symptoms (nausea, vomiting, abdominal distention and pain) while allowing the patient to return home. Additionally the PEG can allow for administration of medications (particularly those used in palliation of symptoms) and for comfort feeds at the end of life. Complications of venting PEGs typically are classified as minor (peristomal leakage, pain at the PEG tube insertion site, insufficient drainage) or major (tube dislodgement, peritonitis). Causes of peristomal leakage include infection, gastric hypersecretion, and torsion of the PEG tube. ED interventions may include relief of external torsion, application of barrier creams, and perhaps addition of antisecretory agents. Insufficient drainage may be corrected with bedside flushing.

In the case of loss of the PEG catheter (whether being used for enteral feeds or for management of an MBO), replacement depends on the age of the catheter track. For gastrostomy sites which are well granulated and have been present for weeks to months, the temporary placement of a small Foley catheter can prevent closure of the stoma as long as the Foley is placed within 24 hours of initial catheter loss. There are potential complications, including the creation of a false passage. Proper placement should be ensured with a radiopaque injection and plain film of the abdomen. If, on the other hand, the catheter is dislodged within 4 weeks of initial placement, patients are at significant risk of peritonitis and perforation due to peritoneal spillage of gastric contents through the immature track. In such cases, replacement should not be attempted without consultation with gastroenterology, interventional radiology, or general surgery. For patients very close to the end of life, there may be more burden than benefit in continuing enteral feedings. In the ED the emergency clinician needs to assess the GOC (does the patient/family want to continue the PEG) and the benefits and burdens of the tube. A conversation regarding the benefits and burdens of enteral feeding could be initiated depending on the patient's clinical condition.

PERIPHERALLY INSERTED CENTRAL CATHETER

PICC lines are commonly used in patients with serious illness to administer support medications such as antibiotics and inotropes, and total parenteral nutrition. Potential complications of PICC lines include dislodgement, infection, thrombosis, and blockage. GOC should be reviewed to assess if the PICC line is necessary to achieve these goals, taking into consideration the patient's clinical status and the benefits and burdens of what is being administered through the PICC line. In heart failure the two most common inotropes prescribed are dobutamine and milrinone. Based on their properties, dobutamine generally must be given via central line (e.g., peripherally inserted central catheter, tunneled line, and port), whereas milrinone may be given via a peripheral line (e.g., peripheral venous catheter and peripheral intravenous line). For patients receiving milrinone or dobutamine who present with complications with their PICC line, the medication can be run through a peripheral IV for a limited time period (typically less than 24 hours), thus giving the ED a way to continue the infusion more easily and may allow for safe discharge if PICC line can be replaced the following day.

LEFT VENTRICULAR ASSIST DEVICES

Treatments for advanced heart failure include both pharmacologic and device management options. Left ventricular assist devices (LVADs) are becoming increasingly common as more clinical centers gain expertise with device implantation. Complications of LVAD therapy include bleeding, infection (systemic or drive line infection), pump thrombosis, right heart failure, device malfunction, and stroke. Patients either have a device implanted that is intended to be temporary while they await heart transplant (so-called bridge to transplant) or that is intended to be permanent (so-called destination therapy). The latter patients are considered to be in a terminal state with heart failure. In most clinical centers that care for patients with LVADs, there are defined protocols for device malfunction which include calling the LVAD technician as well as the heart failure specialist. In patients in catastrophic complications such as massive hemorrhage or stroke, an emergent GOC conversation is warranted to determine next steps from the ED. This conversation should include the cardiologist, the patient/surrogate, the palliative care service, and emergency clinician. Depending on the patient's condition and the GOC, some patients may elect discontinuation of the LVAD in order to pursue a comfort care course which will require the support of the patient's cardiologist and LVAD technician and team.

CASE CONCLUSION

The patient has several indwelling devices—PICC line, pleural drain, and PEG—two of which have some level of malfunction. The patient is most anxious about her PICC line not working because she feels she won't get her "food" and will starve to death. She reports that her shortness of breath is relieved with frequent pleural fluid drainage, and if she doesn't drain it, she becomes symptomatic after a day or two. While she is comfortable now, she worries that she is going to get short of breath soon. GOC conversation is held in the ED after the patient is told that her PICC line must be removed and that her TPN will need to be held for now. While the patient feels she is not gaining weight on the TPN, she feels it is giving her more time, and she would like to see her son graduate from college in the next month. She is hoping to live until then. She understands she has an infection and that TPN may need to be stopped, but she stated that she couldn't handle that thought "just yet" and requested this issue be readdressed the next day. Palliative care is consulted in the ED to assist with the care plan. Based on GOC to focus on life-prolonging therapies, they recommend an intensive care unit admission for sepsis. They will continue to discuss the benefits, burdens, and ability to continue to offer the TPN. You place an interventional pulmonary consultation to help evaluate the best next steps for the effusion management and if patency of the catheter can be achieved before the patient becomes short of breath.

KEY POINTS

- There are numerous devices employed in the setting of advanced illness to palliate symptoms and improve the quality of life.
- Complications of these devices often lead to ED presentation and are most often related to dislodgement, infection, or blockage.
- Minor complications can sometimes be remedied with bedside interventions which can allow a patient to return home.
- Major complications or complications that are burdensome or those that occur very near the end of life are cause to revisit GOC. ED clinician or palliative care consultant should revisit GOC at the earliest possible moment to gain clarity on ED next steps.

Further Reading

1. Narayanan G, Pezeshkmehr A, Venkat S, Guerrero G, Barbery K. Safety and efficacy of the PleurX catheter for the treatment of malignant ascites. *J Palliat Med.* 2014;17(8):906–912.

2. Lui MM, Rhomas R, Lee YCG. Complications of indwelling pleural catheter use and their management. *BMJ Open Resp Res.* 2016;3:e000123.

3. Roberts ME, Melville E, Berrisford RG, Antunes G, Ali NJ. Management of a malignant pleural effusion: British Thoracic Society pleural disease guideline 2010. *Thorax.* 2010;65(Suppl 2):ii32–ii40.

4. Easson AM, Hinshaw DB, Johnson DL. The role of tube feeding and total parenteral nutrition in advanced illness. *J Am Coll Surg.* 2002;194(2):225–228.

5. Buchman AL. Complications of long-term home total parenteral nutrition. *Dig Dis Sci.* 2001;46(1):1–18.

6. Lee A, Lau TN, Yeong KY. Indwelling catheters for the management of malignant ascites. *Support Care Cancer.* 2000;8:493–499.

7. Dittrich A, Schubert B, Kramer M, Lenz F, Kast K. Benefits and risks of a percutaneous endoscopic gastrostomy for decompression in patients with malignant gastrointestinal obstruction. *Support Care Cancer* 2017;25:2849–2856.

8. Schrag SP Sharma R, Jaik NP, Seamon MJ, Lukaszcyk JJ, Martin NK, Hoey BA, Stawicki SP. Complications related to percutaneous endoscopic gastrostomy tubes. *J Gastrointestin Liver Dis.* 2007;16(4):407–418.

9. Malotte K, Saguros A, Groninger H. Continuous cardiac inotropes in patients with end-stage heart failure: An evolving experience. *J Pain Symptom Manag.* 2017;55(1):159–163.

10. Shah R, Shah M, Aleem A. Gastrostomy tube replacement. In *StatPearls.* StatPearls Publishing; 2021. PMID: 29494029.

11 Knocking at the Door

Kirsten G. Engel and Arthur Derse

Case: A 48-year-old man with no past medical history is found collapsed outside in the yard and is nonresponsive. His wife calls the paramedics, and he is found to be in cardiac arrest. He is transported to the emergency department (ED), where advanced cardiac life support (ACLS) measures are in progress. His wife is seated outside the room. The ED nurse asks if the wife can be allowed in the resuscitation room.

What do you do next?

FAMILY PRESENCE DURING RESUSCITATION

Out-of-hospital cardiac arrest is associated with a very poor prognosis for successful resuscitation, and it is worse for survival to discharge, even in a relatively young and healthy patient like the one presented in this case. This devastating event is, unfortunately, all too familiar to both emergency medical services (EMS) and ED providers. Nonetheless, in these grave circumstances, there is unequivocal evidence that rapid and aggressive resuscitative measures provide the best chance for patient survival. At the same time, providers readily recognize that if initial defibrillation fails, their efforts are most often prolonging an inevitable outcome of death. Despite familiarity with these difficult situations, the inclusion of family members during resuscitation proceedings remains a complex and controversial topic.

In this case, the nurse raises the question about whether the wife may be allowed in the resuscitation room. In the acute moment, the medical team needs a clear policy and protocol to guide their decision-making; however, the underlying considerations are anything but simple and straightforward. For this reason, a detailed understanding of this complicated issue is important for all emergency personnel. Numerous factors on the part of the patient and their loved ones, as well as the ED team, must be thoughtfully considered.

As emergency providers, we are deeply committed to providing the best possible care to our patients in the most critical and intense moments. At first glance, we may instinctively fear that, by allowing the patient's wife into the resuscitation room, we may undermine our primary responsibility to our patient and our efforts to save his life. However, it is important to recognize that family witnessed resuscitation (FWR) is not a threat to emergency providers in our delivery of good care, but rather an opportunity to ensure a patient- and family-centered approach even in critical cases like the one presented. In fact, existing research indicates that FWR provides an opportunity to engage and support family members, while also conferring important potential benefits for the patient and medical team. Professional organizations in both emergency medicine and nursing support the practice of FWR and recommend that family members be given this option whenever feasible and appropriate. This scenario provides an opportunity to examine the evolution of acceptance and support of FWR and specifically discuss this practice from the perspectives of the different participants. Several key factors have been identified as important to the success of FWR, including the use of protocols, which can be used to guide implementation of this practice in the ED.

The practice of FWR initially evolved due to discontent and frustration expressed by families of critically ill and dying patients in the 1980s. During this time, family members voiced concerns that they felt helpless and uninformed because they were often ushered out of the patient's room and received inadequate information about their loved ones in these critical moments. Doyle and colleagues at Foote Hospital in Jackson, Michigan, responded to a police officer's request to be present during the resuscitation of a loved one and, subsequently, embarked on a pioneering study in which relatives were allowed to witness resuscitation proceedings while accompanied by a facilitator. The results of this study and another at Parkland Hospital in Texas in the 1990s by Meyers revealed the first evidence of the potential positive effects of this practice. Study participants described that the opportunity to be present during the resuscitation of their loved one reduced the "agony of waiting" and, in turn, lessened feelings of anxiety and helplessness. Moreover, family members expressed that the experience helped them to understand the critical nature of their loved one's condition and the significant effort made by the medical staff to provide the best possible care. Family members also indicated that their presence during the resuscitation proceedings eased their adjustment to the death of their loved one and, in turn, had a positive effect on their grief and bereavement process. As a resounding endorsement of their experiences, nearly all (94%) of the participants at Foote Hospital indicated that they would make the same choice if given the opportunity again. Despite the positive findings from these and several additional studies, significant skepticism about FWR exists due to concerns about potential risks for harm associated with this practice. In the following sections, we will provide insight into these important issues and perceived barriers as we discuss FWR from the perspective of the patient, medical team, and participating family members.

In the setting of critical illness or injury, the most immediate and paramount concern is that the patient receives rapid, high-quality care. Many have voiced concerns that FWR may negatively impact patient care;

however, evidence from numerous studies provides significant reassurance. After the conclusion of the initial study at Foote Hospital, a policy for FWR was implemented in the ED. Nine years of follow-up by Hansen and colleagues revealed no cases in which family members interfered with or disrupted resuscitation proceedings. Similarly, in the Parkland study, nearly all (97%) surveyed healthcare providers indicated that families who were present during resuscitation and invasive procedures demonstrated appropriate behavior which did not impact their ability to deliver care to their patients. In recent years, several studies have specifically examined the impact of FWR on the performance of critical actions (including chest compressions, defibrillation, and pronouncement of death) in both real and simulated settings. The results of these investigations have demonstrated no differences between scenarios with family presence and those without. Notably, in one study, resident physician teams were randomly assigned to three simulated resuscitation scenarios in which (1) family was not present, (2) family was present and quiet, or (3) family was present and demonstrating a clear grief response (i.e., upset and crying). While there were no differences in performance parameters for teams with and without family present, there was a significant delay in the time to the first round of defibrillation for the teams with an overtly grieving family. This finding highlights the importance of screening and preparation of families prior to their participation in FWR, as well as the provision of support during these events. This intervention can ensure that family presence does not result in any harm to the patient through interference, supporting the ethical principles of beneficence (acting for the patient's benefit) and nonmaleficence (avoiding harm). For obvious reasons, it is challenging to assess the preferences and experiences of patients who require resuscitation due to critical illness and injury. Under normal circumstances, the ethical principle of autonomy and the ethical requirement of confidentiality would mean that patients should be asked for permission before family members witness potentially dramatic medical interventions. In an unexpected emergency resuscitation, this is impossible. However, there is evidence to suggest that most patients perceive benefits from having their family members present during these moments. In an ED study, general patients were asked about their preferences regarding FWR, based on a hypothetical scenario of critical resuscitation, and 72% indicated that they would want to have family present during their care. A few other studies have involved interviewing or surveying survivors of resuscitation events and have found that the majority of these patients prefer having their loved ones with them during these procedures. In particular, patients express that the presence of family members is comforting and may even impact their outcomes, as conveyed in a poignant anecdote from a 60-year-old survivor of cardiac arrest who stated that he was "very much aware of his wife's presence, which was enough of an encouragement for him to continue his fight for survival."[1] Thus, ethical the principle of autonomy (what the patient would want under the circumstances) is supported for the majority of patients by FWR.

Considerations regarding the ED team are paramount. Given the inherent complexity of managing critically ill patients, it is not surprising that the practice of FWR has raised significant concerns among healthcare providers regarding its potential to negatively impact the ED team. Resuscitation in the acute setting is a high-stakes and dynamic endeavor in which providers are rapidly thrust into the process of caring for a critically ill patient with whom they may have no prior relationship. In these moments, providers are also aware that there is a significant and, in some cases, nearly certain risk that their patient will die. As a result, providers face additional challenges due to the emotionally fraught aspects of these encounters with responsibilities to support surviving family members. Even under the best of circumstances these encounters are stressful, but research evidence clearly indicates that the presence of family during resuscitation proceedings does not increase self-reported stress symptoms among providers. Moreover, despite significant fears that FWR may lead to misunderstandings and, in turn, result in increased malpractice litigation, such correlation has not been reported. For providers, the practice of FWR can humanize the resuscitation process by making the team aware of the patient in the larger and important context of their family and loved ones. In moments where healthcare providers realize that efforts to save their patient are failing, they need to transition from treating the patient to now focus on the surviving family members. This process has the opportunity to occur seamlessly when loved ones are present in the resuscitation room; in fact, many healthcare providers who have had experience with FWR will share anecdotes in which family members recognize the futility of further intervention even before the medical team makes the decision to stop. When death is declared, it is clear to all who are present that everything possible has been done to try to "save" the patient. Family members who witness this intense effort have a lower risk of developing guilt, which can complicate the bereavement process. In this way, providers who allow family members to be present during resuscitation actually help these survivors to take the first, critical step in the normal grieving process.

Debriefing sessions following the death of a patient in the ED are a vital intervention as these interactions can facilitate healthy coping and provide opportunities for team members to support one another. In the setting of FWR, debriefing can help providers to reflect on the impact of the experience and provide an important foundation for future resuscitations witnessed by loved ones. Existing research on FWR clearly demonstrates that education, training, and experience play an important role in provider attitudes toward this practice. Numerous studies reveal an increasing gradient of support for FWR, dependent on years of clinical practice and previous experience with having family members present during resuscitation procedures. In the following statement, a trauma surgeon describes the dramatic change in his views toward FWR, after allowing a family to be present during the resuscitation of their young daughter: "I had previously opposed any intrusion into the sacred domain of the trauma resuscitation room by patients' families. I now realize that under the proper circumstances . . . the presence of the family may actually be a good thing for everyone, including the caregivers."[2]

Since its beginning, the primary focus of FWR has been its potential to benefit the families of patients who are facing sudden, life-threatening illness or injury. Extensive evidence indicates that FWR serves to engage, inform, and empower family members so that they are better prepared to understand and accept abrupt, often heartbreaking changes, in the health of a loved one. For more than three decades, FWR has been practiced with variable frequency in different medical settings, including intensive care units, inpatient cardiac wards, and the ED. However, the widespread dissemination and adoption of this practice have been hindered, in part, by concerns that FWR may also cause psychological harm to participating families. During resuscitation efforts, family members are inevitably exposed to potentially upsetting images or disturbing interventions involving the care of their loved one. While no negative sequelae were observed during the initial studies at Foote and Parkland Hospitals, it is only in recent years that significant research has directly explored rates of psychological trauma and, specifically posttraumatic stress disorder (PTSD), following FWR. In 2011, Compton et al. published a prospective comparison study which demonstrated no difference in PTSD and depression scores for family members who witnessed resuscitation (active CPR) in the ED and those who did not.[3] A larger randomized controlled study by Jabre et al. found reduced rates of PTSD and better long-term grief outcomes (1 year) among family members in the intervention group, who were given the opportunity to witness prehospital CPR, as compared to the control group, who were not given this option.[4,5] These results suggest that FWR actually may be a protective factor for families who are present during the care of life-threatening illness in a loved one. Additional research is needed to better understand if this positive effect is also present in hospital settings, but clearly, there appears to be no evidence to suggest that FWR contributes to worse outcomes for participants.

A detailed understanding of the impact of FWR on patients, the ED team, and families serves as an essential foundation for identifying the factors which are important for successful implementation of this practice. There are numerous key factors for the success of FWR implementation (see Box 11.1).

FWR should be always be presented to families as an option, and it is important that family members are given the choice to accept or decline this opportunity. Some individuals will prefer not to be present during resuscitation activities of their loved one, and this choice should be accepted and supported.

BOX 11.1 **Factors for Success in Family Witnessed Resuscitation**

- Family witnessed resuscitation as an option
- Family member screening
- Family support person
- Family witnessed resuscitation policy and protocol
- Staff education and training
- Debriefing

All family members should be screened. Before family members are given the option for FWR, they should be screened by an experienced member of the ED staff (e.g., nursing, social work) for emotional instability, combative behavior, intoxication, or altered mental status. If these elements are evident, family members should be excluded from FWR.

There should always be a family support person. A member of the ED staff should be assigned to support the family during FWR and should remain with them throughout their experience. This family support person should be familiar with typical resuscitation activities so that they can provide families with explanations and clarifications as desired. In addition, they should help the family to know where they can stand so that they do not interfere with care delivery but have the opportunity for contact with the patient when possible and desired. Last, the family support person should be prepared to support a healthy process of grief and bereavement for the family.

There should be a FWR policy and protocol in place. An established departmental policy and accompanying protocol for FWR are essential to ensure that expectations, procedures, and responsibilities are clear for all participating staff in the acute setting of resuscitation (Box 11.2).

The staff require education and training. The success of FWR is critically dependent on the education, training, and experience of ED staff. Department-specific policies are needed to establish expectations and norms of care regarding the role of FWR. This is particularly helpful for new or transient members of the emergency care team. Protocols provide specific parameters for "how" FWR will be carried out in the ED. Prior to implementing a policy and protocol for FWR in the ED, it is important to provide staff education and training. Role play is a valuable teaching approach and should be considered for staff training. Clinicians who have prior experience with FWR can also be helpful in providing insight and support to others during training.

Offer debriefing after an episode of family witnessed resuscitation. After any death in the ED, it is important to have an opportunity for staff debriefing, but this is particularly critical in situations in which family has been present. FWR intensifies awareness among ED staff of the social and emotional significance of the patient's death, and debriefing sessions can help to support healthy coping for ED providers.

BOX 11.2 Sample Family Witnessed Resuscitation Policy and Protocol

Policy: Whenever possible, family members will be given the option to be present in the patient care area of the emergency department (ED) during the resuscitation of their loved one.

Purpose: To provide families with the opportunity to be with their loved one in the event of critical injury or illness, while ensuring the highest quality of care for our patients.

1. All potential visiting family members will be screened by an experienced member of ED staff for emotional instability, combative behavior, intoxication, and altered mental status. Exclusions will be made in circumstances of clear and compelling evidence of inappropriate behavior. Every effort will be made to provide this option to as many families as possible.
2. Prior to escorting the family into the resuscitation room, a family support person (FSP) will inform the ED staff caring for the patient of the family's desire to be present. If the ED and/or trauma staff agree that visitation is possible and appropriate, the patient's wishes for family presence will be assessed (in the event that the patient is conscious). Provided that all are in agreement, the family will be given the option to be present in the resuscitation area.
3. The option of FWR will be given to no more than two family members at a time. Any family member who declines this option will be supported in their decision and will continue to receive frequent updates on the status of their loved one during ongoing resuscitation.
4. Family members will be accompanied by a FSP in the resuscitation area at all times. In the event of more than one critical resuscitation occurring simultaneously, the opportunity for FWR will be based on availability of additional staff to serve in the role as FSP. In the resuscitation area, the FSP will help to explain the patient's appearance, team activities, and room equipment, as well as answer questions. Depending on the circumstances, the resident, attending physician, or nurse may help to provide some additional information to the family during the events of the resuscitation.
5. Family members will be given the opportunity to touch the patient or hold their foot or hand, as the circumstances of the resuscitation allow. If feasible and appropriate, family members will be encouraged to speak out loud to their loved one while in the resuscitation room.
6. Any family member demonstrating inappropriate, distracting, or excessively emotional behavior will be immediately escorted out of the room by the FSP. At any time, the attending emergency

medicine or trauma physician may request that the family's visit be terminated.

7. In the event of death of the patient, the family will be taken back to the private room by the FSP with reassurance that they will have the opportunity to return to see their loved one once preparations have been made for all of the family to come in.

CASE CONCLUSION

In this vignette, the nurse's question asks us to consider the needs of family members while engaged in the challenging task of caring for a critically ill patient with a high likelihood of death. In these difficult and humbling moments, our obligations to our patient should be balanced with our responsibility to loved ones who are facing immense stress and often heartbreaking loss. Allowing a family member to be present during a resuscitation not only has the potential to benefit the included individual and their subsequent bereavement process but also has positive implications for ED providers and patients themselves. While there is strong evidence to support this practice, its successful implementation requires a thoughtful process of preparation and planning. Specifically, both a department-specific policy and protocol are essential to establish clear expectations and guide practice. Moreover, provider training and ongoing support for participants are also key components. Above all, it is important to recognize that such changes in practice require time and patience, but ultimately enable us to further our commitment to providing both patient- and family-centered care.

KEY POINTS

- FWR may reduce the risk of PTSD for participating family members and help to ensure a healthy grieving process in the event of patient death.
- It is very important to establish a policy and protocol regarding FWR in your department. Consider offering families the option to be present during resuscitation events whenever feasible and appropriate.

- Education, training, and experience with FWR are key factors influencing provider support for this practice. While opposition and skepticism are common, opportunities to learn about and experience FWR often change provider attitudes.
- During FWR, participating family members should receive adequate support and have the opportunity to touch or speak with their loved one when possible.

Further Reading

1. Belanger MA, Reed S. A rural community hospital's experience with family-witnessed resuscitation. *Journal of Emergency Nursing.* 1997 Jun;23(3):238–239. doi:10.1016/s0099-1767(97)90015-5. PMID: 9283361.
2. Barone JE. Family presence during trauma resuscitation. *Journal of Trauma.* 2001 Feb;50(2):386. doi:10.1097/00005373-200102000-00034. PMID: 11242312.
3. Compton S, Levy P, Griffin M, Waselewsky D, Mango LM, Zalenski R. Family-witnessed resuscitation: Bereavement outcomes in an urban environment. *Journal of Palliative Medicine.* 2011;14(6):715–721.
4. Jabre P, Belpomme V, Azoulay E, Jacob L, Bertrand L, et al. Family presence during cardiopulmonary resuscitation. *NEJM.* 2013;368:1008–1018.
5. Jabre P, Tazarourte K, Azoulay E, Borron SW, Belpomme V, Jacob L, et al. Offering the opportunity for family to be present during cardiopulmonary resuscitation. *Intensive Care Med.* 2014;40:981–987.
6. Doyle CJ, Post H, Burney RE, Maino J, Keefe M, Rhee KJ. Family participation during resuscitation: An option. *Annals of Emergency Medicine.* 1987;16:s673–675.
7. Hanson C, Strawser D. Family presence during cardiopulmonary resuscitation: Foote Hospital emergency department's nine-year perspective. *Journal of Emergency Nursing.* 1992;18:104–106.
8. Robinson SM, Mackenzie-Ross S, Campbell Hewson GL, Egleston CV, Prevost AT. Psychological effect of witnessed resuscitation on bereaved relatives. *Lancet.* 1998;352:614–617.
9. Meyers TA, Eichhorn DJ, Guzzetta CE, et al. Family presence during invasive procedures and resuscitation. *American Journal of Nursing.* 2000;100:32–42.
10. Eichhorn DJ, Meyers TA, Guzzetta CE, et al. Family presence during invasive procedures and resuscitation: Hearing the voice of the patient. *American Journal of Nursing.* 2001;101:48–55.
11. Sacchetti A, Paston C, Carraccio C. Family members do not disrupt care when present during invasive procedures. *AEM.* 2005;12(5):477–479.

12. Fernandez R, Compton S, Jones KA, Velilla MA. The presence of a family witness impacts physician performance during simulated medical codes. *Crit Care Med.* 2009;37(6):1956–1960.

13. Engel KG, Barnosky AR, Berry-Bovia M, Desmond JS, Ubel PA. Provider experience and attitudes toward family presence during resuscitation procedures. *Journal of Palliative Medicine.* 2007;10(5):1007–1009.

14. Porter JE, Cooper SJ, Sellick K. Family presence during resuscitation (FPDR): Perceived benefits, barriers and enablers to implementation and practice. *International Emergency Nursing.* 2013;22:69–74.

15. Flanders SA, Strasen JH. Review of evidence about family presence during resuscitation. *Crit Care Nurs Clin North.* 2014;26:533–550.

16. Oczkowski SJW, Mazzetti I, Cupido C, Fox-Robichaud AE. Family presence during resuscitation: A Canadian Critical Care Society position paper. *Can Respir Journal.* 2015;22(4):201–205.

17. Johnson C. A literature review examining barriers to implementation of family witnessed resuscitation in the emergency department. *International Emergency Nursing.* 2017;30:31–35.

12 "Take It Off . . . Now"

Ashley Shreves

Case: An 85-year-old man presents to the emergency department (ED) with acute onset of altered mental status. He is unresponsive on arrival with a Glascow Coma Score of 3. His blood glucose is normal. He is intubated immediately. Computer tomography of the brain is performed, and he is found to have a massive intracerebral hemorrhage with signs of impending herniation. His bleed is inoperable, and his overall prognosis is poor. You and the neurosurgeon meet with his wife to discuss goals of care. Best- and worst-case scenarios are discussed, and the patient's wife ultimately decides to forgo further life-extending interventions for her husband. The wife asks that he be removed from life support in the ED and be allowed to die.

What do you do now?

"TAKE IT OFF . . . NOW"

In this case, there is a request for removal of life-sustaining treatment (LST) after its initiation. Typical reasons for this in the ED include (1) goals-of-care change after more clinical information becomes available and/or (2) there is an advance care plan (through discussion and or documentation) previously unknown or recognized that LSTs were not or are no longer wanted based on a patient's known illness trajectory.

Emergency providers are highly skilled in the practice of airway management and the initiation of mechanical ventilation. Mechanical ventilation is a type of LST that can be a vital tool in supporting patients through critical illness. In some patients, however, particularly those living with an advanced and/or terminal illness, the use of LST, like mechanical ventilation, can be burdensome and harmful. In select patients, these kinds of support devices can be "bridges to nowhere," artificially prolonging the patient's dying process in a way that is neither helpful nor desired. Knowing when and how to discontinue mechanical ventilation is a necessary skill. This process has traditionally been termed a "terminal extubation," though in some institutions, alternative language such as "palliative extubation" and "ventilator liberation" are recommended. While there is considerable education about the indications for intubating a patient in the ED, there is little education about the indications for ventilator withdrawal and the appropriate method for managing this procedure.

Patients commonly engage in advance care planning and complete advance directives to communicate their wishes about the use of LST and end-of-life care. Unfortunately, it has been well-demonstrated that advance directives do not always travel with patients. Even when advance directives have been completed, emergency providers have difficulty accessing these documents within the electronic medical record. In addition, clinical information that could guide end-of-life decision-making is often incomplete in the first minutes of a patient's ED presentation, making it challenging for patients and families to make decisions about withholding life-sustaining interventions. Understandably, physicians often err on the side of providing LST until more information is available—whether it be in the form of clinical data or advance directives. Once more information is available, however, it may become clear that continuing with mechanical ventilation is inconsistent with the patient's expressed wishes, goals, and values, particularly in the context of a devastating illness that carries a poor prognosis. Goals such as comfort, avoiding suffering, and being allowed to die naturally may supersede the desire to simply live longer. In this case, it is appropriate to withdraw mechanical ventilation and other interventions or support devices and allow the patient to die from his or her underlying disease process. From a legal and ethical perspective, withholding and withdrawing LST are generally considered equivalent. Courts have upheld the right of patients and their surrogate decision makers to withdraw LST based on the principle of patient autonomy and the right of informed refusal. The specific rules and procedures that inform the withdrawal of mechanical ventilation may vary across states and institutions.

Communication is critical. As would be the case in any major decision about withholding or withdrawing LST, a thorough and comprehensive discussion between provider and surrogate decision-maker outlining the patient's goals of care should transpire before any action is taken. Families and/or surrogate decision makers typically find making decisions about withdrawing LST incredibly stressful. Families often have the mistaken impression that they are deciding whether the patient lives or dies, and the burden of that responsibility can feel emotionally overwhelming. Most commonly, when withdrawal is being considered, death is inevitable and the ventilator is serving as a means of artificially prolonging the patient's dying process. Conceptually reframing this for families can be enormously helpful in allowing them to move forward with this decision. It is also critically important to avoid the phrase "withdrawal of care," as it can give the mistaken impression that the patient is being abandoned. Instead, care is being "transitioned" from focusing on life prolongation to focusing on comfort and supporting the patient through a natural dying process. Alternately, it can be said that the patient is being "liberated" from machines and other devices so that he or she can have a natural death.

MECHANICAL VENTILATION WITHDRAWAL PROCEDURE

In all cases, before any withdrawal procedure begins, a meeting with the legal surrogate should occur that includes the legal surrogate, any other family members, and the interdisciplinary team available to support in the

ED (such as chaplain, social worker, palliative care team members). In this meeting, the clinician leading the removal of LST should (1) confirm the goals of care, (2) explain the procedure and what will be done, (3) explain the role of medications, (4) establish any important rituals or ceremonies that they would like, (5) establish who will be in the room during the procedure, and (6) establish expectations regarding survival with a statement such as "They may live minutes, hours, or days."

There is some debate about the process for ventilator withdrawal (Table 12.1). Some advocate for a "terminal weaning" process whereby the amount of ventilatory support is gradually reduced and then ultimately removed. Alternatively, the endotracheal tube is abruptly removed. A recent prospective study comparing the two methods found no difference in surrogate psychological distress at 3 months, the primary outcome, between groups. Those patients undergoing immediate extubation, however, did experience more airway obstruction and gasping and exhibited more signs of overall discomfort. If a terminal weaning process is desired, the oxygen level and positive pressure should be gradually decreased, over roughly 30 minutes, while opioids are titrated to match the patient's symptom burden. The patient's code status should be updated to Do Not Resuscitate (DNR) if the decision is made to move forward with a palliative extubation. *Attention to spiritual health and faith traditions is important.* It should be determined whether the patient is from a faith background to ensure that their spiritual needs can be met prior to death, when possible. Many hospitals have chaplains available that can be summoned to the bedside to offer prayer and/or particular end-of-life rituals important to families from certain religious communities.

The primary symptoms to anticipate and control in ventilator withdrawal are dyspnea and anxiety. There is considerable variation in the severity of this symptom across patients, with those patients extubated after a devastating neurologic event and/or coma exhibiting less dyspnea than those with other underlying diagnoses like sepsis and multiorgan failure. This patient population is generally unable to verbally communicate their level of discomfort, so nonverbal signs of dyspnea such as gasping, accessory muscle use, and tachypnea should be assessed and monitored. Use of a validated scale for respiratory distress such as the Respiratory Distress Observation Scale (RDOS) is recommended.

TABLE 12.1 **Key Steps in Ventilator Withdrawal**

Key Steps	Details
1. Confirm	Confirm request and recommendations for removal of life-sustaining therapy (LST).
2. Goal of Care/Surrogate Information	Perform a goals-of-care discussion with legal surrogate decision-makers and if goals confirm removal of LST in the emergency department: (1) explain the procedure and what will be done, (2) explain the role of medications, (3) establish any important rituals or ceremonies that they would like, (4) establish who will be in the room during the procedure, and (5) establish expectations regarding survival with a statement such as "they may live minutes, hours, or days after removal of the ventilator."
3. Do-Not-Resuscitate (DNR) Order	Ensure DNR order is written before process begins
4. Environment/Resources	Tend to the environment: turn off monitors, bring in chairs; determine who will be in the room and where they will be; ensure availability of nurses, medications, and support.
5. Spiritual/Rituals	Ensure spiritual needs are met and rituals complete.
6. Pre-Extubation Simulation	Perform spontaneous breathing trial; assess symptoms (dyspnea and anxiety/agitation). If significant symptoms, administer small bolus of opiate and/or benzodiazepine.
7. Titrate	Titrate down vent support, administering appropriate medications to maintain comfort.
8. Extubate	Remove endotracheal tube (have chuck pad and suction ready for cleaning).
9. Symptom Control	Reassess symptoms and titrate medications accordingly. Consider starting opiate infusion if needing frequent redosing of medication.
10. Death Disclosure/After-Death Care	If the patient dies in the emergency department, the clinician should perform a death disclosure and ensure there is aftercare by support team.

Pre-extubation simulation is recommended. To estimate the amount of respiratory distress that the patient might experience prior to extubation, a breathing trial while on the ventilator might be helpful. Turn the ventilator to a spontaneous mode with pressure support while watching carefully to avoid desaturation; this will allow an estimation of the amount of distress that the patient might have, once extubated. If the patient exhibits distress, it is important to return the ventilator to full support and begin appropriate medications to mitigate distress followed by serial tests. A comfortable rate of spontaneous breathing, if the patient's condition allows for this, is the goal. When using medications for dyspnea, the goal is comfort, not apnea.

Prior to endotracheal tube (ETT) removal, the tape and/or ETT holder should be disconnected and the balloon cuff deflated. A protective pad should be placed over the patient's chest to "catch" the ETT and protect the patient's gown from the inevitable secretions, some of which may be bloody. The ETT and any other invasive tubes should then be pulled out and discarded.

In patients who breathe spontaneously during a breathing trial, opioids are the first-line agents for palliating dyspnea after an extubation. Prior to extubation, a bolus dose is generally administered. If morphine is the agent of choice, an appropriate dose ranges from 2 to 6 mg IV, in opioid-naïve patients. Equi-ananalgesic equivalents of hydromophone and fentanyl can safely be used for this purpose. After initial bolus dosing, the easiest way to rapidly and effectively titrate opioids to alleviate dyspnea is to use a continuous opioid infusion, if available. Once off the ventilator, the amount of morphine needed to ensure patient comfort varies, but in one study, the average amount needed in the last hour of life was 11 mg. Repeat opioid boluses are frequently needed in the minutes following ventilator withdrawal, particularly if a weaning process is not used. As mentioned above, nonverbal signs of dyspnea such as gasping, tachypnea, and accessory muscle use should be assessed and used as a guide when titrating opioids. An initial infusion can start at 4–10 mg/hour but may need to be rapidly titrated to match individual patient needs. While providers may have concerns about causing respiratory depression and death with opioids, in one study there was a direct relationship between opioid dosing and time to death, with those patients receiving higher opioid doses actually living longer (Table 12.2).

Patients in the last hours of life commonly exhibit noisy breathing, colloquially known as the death rattle. Anecdotally, this symptom is almost

TABLE 12.2 **Key Medications for Ventilator Withdrawal**

Medication	Initial dose (bolus) with redose every 10 minutes if needed; infusions should only be initiated once comfort is attained from bolus.
Opioids	
Morphine	2–4 mg
Hydromorphone	0.2–0.6 mg
Fentanyl	50–100 μg
Benzodiazepines	
Lorazepam	1–2 mg
Midazolam	1–2 mg
Diazepam	5–10 mg

universally present in patients after a palliative extubation. The etiology of this symptom is multifactorial. Glycopyrrolate and atropine are commonly administered prior to ventilator withdrawal in an attempt to dry up patient secretions and thus lessen the sound made by pooled secretions in the oropharynx. The evidence for this intervention is weak. Patient repositioning can be effective. Reassurance to family members about the lack of patient discomfort associated with this symptom is often the most important intervention.

When anxiety is assessed and anticipated with or without respiratory distress, many patients in addition to opioids will require benzodiazepines. Lorazepam and midazolam are reasonable agents to consider. As with opiates, some patients should actually receive a small bolus dose of these medications prior to ventilator removal, if there are signs of agitation with the spontaneous breathing trial. If agitation and/or anxiety continue post tube removal, additional bolus doses can be administered. Patients rarely need a continuous benzodiazepine infusion.

While some patients are transitioned from the ventilator to a supplemental oxygen delivery device such as a nonrebreather or nasal cannula, this step is unnecessary and patients can generally be extubated to room air. Opioids can more effectively palliate dyspnea than oxygen. Furthermore, the use of oxygen can artificially prolong the patient's dying process without adding to comfort.

TIME TO DEATH/PROGNOSIS

Education regarding estimated time to death is an important factor. It is important to prepare family members and loved ones for the expected trajectory of patients undergoing a palliative extubation. It can be challenging to predict how long someone will live off the ventilator. For this reason, family members should be prepared for a range of possibilities. Some patients die minutes after ventilator withdrawal while others live for days. It is easier to prognosticate once the ventilator has been removed and the patient's respiratory effort and ability to oxygenate can be assessed. In one intensive care unit (ICU) study, average time to death after extubation was between 2 and 3 hours. Typical guidance would be that "Your family member could live minutes, hours, or days. We will know more after we remove the ventilator."

DISPOSITION

Patients expected to die within minutes to hours should generally not have to experience the burdens of a care setting transfer. Their dying process and death can and should be managed within the ED. Efforts should be made to create a peaceful and comfortable space for the patient and family, bringing in chairs, turning off monitors and alarms, for instance. For those patients with relatively stable vital signs and an anticipated prognosis of hours to days, several disposition options exist. Where and when available, it is preferable to enroll patients in hospice care to ensure they receive expert management of their end-of-life symptoms. Hospice care is delivered in both the inpatient and home setting. Most patients post palliative extubation, particularly those on opioid infusions, qualify for inpatient hospice care. Patients with highly motivated and competent caregivers may even be able to return home, under the care and guidance of hospice.

CASE CONCLUSION

For the patient in this vignette, goals of care were clearly established by his wife as comfort and removal from LST in the ED. A spontaneous breathing trial was performed, and he had no spontaneous respirations, no facial grimacing, or other signs of distress. Based on this assessment, no medications were required prior to extubation. His wife requested that their only daughter be present. One dose of glycopyrollate was given 15 minutes prior to extubation. After assessing for spiritual needs, a chaplain was offered and at the bedside at the time of extubation. Family meeting was held with the patient's wife and daughter to tell them what to expect before, during, and after the extubation. He was moved out of the resuscitation room to a private room, where he was extubated and died 10 minutes after extubation.

KEY POINTS

- Ventilator withdrawal occurs in the ED, and the request should be honored whenever appropriate.
- A careful goals-of-care discussion that incorporates prognostic data and patient values and goals is necessary before moving forward with ventilator withdrawal.
- There is no fixed dose of medication for this procedure. Some patients will need little to no medication to manage the transition off ventilator. Others will need opiates and benzodiazepines, given as a bolus and infusion.
- Medications should be administered based on object distress scales.
- When administering medications, a comfortable breathing pattern and the absence of agitation/anxiety are the goals, not respiratory depression.

Further Reading

1. Robert R, Le Gouge A, Kentish-Barnes N, et al. Terminal weaning or immediate extubation for withdrawing mechanical ventilation in critically ill patients (the ARREVE observational study). *Intensive Care Med.* 2017;43:1793–1807.
2. Huynh TN, Walling AM, Le TX, et al. Factors associated with palliative withdrawal of mechanical ventilation and time to death after withdrawal. *J Palliat Med.* 2013;16:1368–1374.
3. Mazer MA, Alligood CM, Wu Q. The infusion of opioids during terminal withdrawal of mechanical ventilation in the medical intensive care unit. *J Pain Symptom Manage.* 2011;42:44–51.

4. Campbell ML, Templin T, Walch J. A respiratory distress observation scale for patients unable to self-report dyspnea. *J Palliat Med.* 2010;13:285–289.
5. O'Mahony S, McHugh M, Zallman L, et al. Ventilator withdrawal: Procedures and outcomes. Report of a collaboration between a critical care division and a palliative care service. *J Pain Symptom Manage.* 2003;26:954–961.
6. Campbell ML, Yarandi HN, Mendez M. A two-group trial of a terminal ventilator withdrawal algorithm: Pilot testing. *J Palliat Med.* 2015;18:781–785.
7. Delannoy TD, Robineau O, Meybeck A, et al. Comparison of terminal extubation and terminal weaning as mechanical ventilation withdrawal in ICU patients. *Minverva Anestesiol.* 2017;83:375–382.
8. Welie JV, Ten Have HA. The ethics of forgoing life-sustaining treatment: Theoretical considerations and clinical decision making. *Multidiscip Respir Med.* 2014;9:14.
9. Campbell ML. How to withdraw mechanical ventilation: A systematic review of the literature. *AACN Adv Crit Care.* 2007;18:397–403.
10. Epker JL, Bakker J, Kompanje EJO. The use of opioids and sedatives and time until death after withdrawing mechanical ventilation and vasoactive drugs in a Dutch intensive care unit. *Anesth Analg* 2011;112:628–634.

13 Judgment Awaits

Joanne Kuntz

Case: A 2-month-old girl presents to the
emergency department (ED) in cardiac arrest.
Her parents report that they placed the child in
her crib in a supine position 2 hours prior to
discovering her limp and blue in her crib. They
immediately called 911. Emergency medical
services (EMS) reports that on arrival the parents
were attempting cardiopulmonary resuscitation
(CPR). EMS confirmed the infant was without
pulse or respirations and initiated advanced
cardiac life support. On arrival to the ED, she
is intubated with CPR in progress with the
parents in the room. After 15 minutes, there is
no return of spontaneous circulation. The baby is
pronounced dead in the ED.

What do you do now?

PEDIATRIC DEATH IN THE EMERGENCY DEPARTMENT

Annually, there are 55,000 pediatric deaths in the United States (CDC 2010); with over 1,100 EDs (Emergency Department Benchmarking Alliance), this means that despite the relative infrequency of pediatric death, among emergency medicine providers, exposure to pediatric death is surprisingly common. The acuity, prematurity, and gravity of pediatric mortality complicate the bereavement process for providers and parents. In 2019, there were about 3,400 cases of sudden unexpected infant death (SUID) and 342 unexplained deaths in children (1–18 years) in the United States (https://www.cdc.gov/sids/data.htm). SUID occurs among infants less than 12 months and has no immediately obvious cause (https://www.cdc.gov/sids/data.htm). Many providers may be familiar with the term "sudden infant death syndrome" (SIDS). SUID includes SIDS (37%), accidental suffocation in a sleeping environment (28.3%), and other deaths from unknown causes (34.3%) (https://www.cdc.gov/sids/about/index.htm). Additionally, sudden unexplained death in childhood (SUDC) describes unexplained deaths in children between 1 and 18 years (https://sudc.org/facts-statistics/). These types of sudden pediatric deaths are considered unexplained after a review of the clinical history and circumstances of death, and performance of a complete autopsy with appropriate ancillary testing fail to determine cause of death. SUID is more common than SUDC (90.1 deaths per 100,000 live births vs. 1.0–1.4 deaths per 100,000 of the population). Both SUID and SUDC are more common in American Indian/Alaska Native and Non-Hispanic Blacks compared to Non-Hispanic Whites (https://www.cdc.gov/sids/data.htm).[1]

SUDC places families at high risk for complicated bereavement. All ages are affected by loss; the specific impact and conceptualization of death vary by cognitive capacity and developmental stage, which is important to consider when offering support to parents as well as siblings of the patient. The process of addressing this should begin prior to death pronouncement with attention to family presence during resuscitation.

Although the tendency is to exclude caregivers from the resuscitation efforts, the data investigating both the barriers and the benefits of this exposure encourage a different approach.[2] Anecdotally, providers report fear of litigious ramifications, obstruction of care, and traumatization of caregivers as barriers to inviting caregivers to witness resuscitation. Contrary to this notion, recent studies have elucidated that family presence during resuscitation allows them to feel that everything has been done, to process more concretely what has happened, and to have the opportunity to offer comfort to their child, all of which mitigate complicated bereavement.[3] Situations that may pose more ethical anguish are when to terminate resuscitation efforts and when to not initiate them at all (specifically in the realm of premature birth).

The sudden and unexpected nature of death described in this case adds additional complexity in that this is a reportable death and will require the physician and medical team to balance compassionate care for the family with their obligate forensic responsibilities and cooperation with the local investigating authorities. Additionally, it is often impossible to determine whether a potentially lethal condition has resulted from intentional or accidental causes. The healthcare team should refrain from speculating on the cause of death when a medicolegal investigation is pending. While this may feel supportive, it often undermines the relationship with the investigating authorities who are legally charged with determining the cause of death and adds unnecessary stress for the family when the healthcare team and legal authorities are in disagreement (https://sudc.org/research-medical-info/medical-care-after-sudc).

Developing prior agreements or memoranda of understanding with your local chief medicolegal death investigation officer will allow ED staff to clearly communicate with families what services they have to offer while at the ED, versus what the medical examiner/coroner or funeral home can also provide to ensure smooth collaboration between agencies, protection of forensic evidence, the collection of bio-specimens, and compassionate care of the family.

Time, space, and privacy to be with the child's body after death are often overlooked in the whirl of the ED setting, but they can be easily accommodated and significantly beneficial for the grieving parent.[4] Although typically relegated to large pediatric centers with a devoted child life specialist, legacy making can be easily incorporated into any setting. In this digital age, smart phones provide easy access to photography; pictures of loved ones holding hands with the child offer a non-gruesome way to commemorate a bond. Similarly, when permitted by the local investigating authority, hand and footprints or a lock of hair can be meaningful tokens.

With any pediatric death, providing the opportunity for the family to view the body is another key component that affects bereavement. Not only does it allow an opportunity to say goodbye for parents, but it also helps young siblings who may want to visit to anchor the reality of the situation and preclude imagined visions of the patient (which are often more traumatizing than reality), in accordance with their developmental stage (see Box 13.1). It is also important to honor the family's preference should they decline the opportunity. Prior to viewing and with the approval of local death investigating authorities, it is helpful to describe what the family might see and to cover (but not remove) any medical devices, wounds, or bodily fluids that may cause additional distress. Ideally, the family should be afforded unlimited and private time with the body, with multiple viewings, if requested.[5] In some institutions, pediatric patients do not go to the morgue but are transferred directly to the funeral home, which allows for additional time for the family to spend time with their child. Establishing memoranda of understanding with local investigative authorities in advance of such cases allows for efficient care and communication.

Bereavement is a process and will continue long after the next of kin leave the emergency room; having resources for ongoing support and

---

BOX 13.1 **Key Steps for Sudden Infant Death in the Emergency Department**

1. Ensure protocols in place for sudden unexplained death in childhood (SUDC) that are developed in conjunction with local death-investigating authorities.
2. Establish a protocol for family presence surrounding pediatric resuscitative efforts and postmortem visitation, with careful consideration of interdisciplinary support such as social work and chaplaincy.
3. Build a repertoire of supplies to afford legacy-making opportunities at the bedside.
4. Dedicate a team member (chaplain, social worker, nurse) who will ensure provision of follow-up resources to family prior to emergency department departure and/or facilitate phone call to family for additional support.
5. Construct time and space to accommodate a debriefing session with all participating staff.

---

follow-up with families after a death is critical to how families navigate their grief. Given that this piece may not be appropriate to address in the acute situation, it can be helpful to provide a list of counseling resources and bereavement groups to families before leaving the hospital. When possible, having a dedicated person to follow up in the subsequent days to weeks is also helpful. Leveraging the skills of other members of your team such as chaplains, social workers, child-life therapists, and psychologists, when available, ensures attention to all aspects of care—social, emotional, spiritual, and psychological.

Although there is rarely a quiet moment in the ED, it is important to protect time and space to acknowledge the effect of a child's death on staff. This remains important to the health of the individual staff member but also to the effectiveness of the team—the ability to continue caring for other patients who need care. This may look like a prayer or mantra at the end of a code or a more formal debriefing session. It is also important to notify key providers (i.e., pediatrician) who have cared for the patient prior to the death if they are not present and encourage parents or guardians to schedule a follow-up appointment. Families expect that their primary care provider will be aware of their child's death, and the task of notifying them of the child's team should not fall to the family. Ideally, the primary care team should reach out to the bereaved parents/guardians to arrange for a follow-up visit,[6] but if the family has no primary care provider, then it is crucial that ED follow up to ensure applicable resources are provided and referrals made.

The death of a child in the ED is one of the most challenging problems facing emergency healthcare providers.[6] Any pediatric death is difficult and when they occur unexpectedly and without immediate explanation, they can be extremely difficult. Although relatively rare events, all ED providers should be aware of the prevalence of both SUID and SUDC and be prepared to care for both the patient and surviving family members. The complexity of these cases highlights the need for an interdisciplinary approach that includes many different members of the emergency care team. Pre-existing relationships with investigating authorities can help to ensure a collaborative effort that preserves both the rights of the bereaved family affected by this tragedy and the physical evidence when there is concern for accidental or intentional injury. The death of a child is a critical incident;

honoring the life of the deceased child and the efforts of all staff involved with a simple communal mantra that recognizes the life of the child and gratitude for the work of the staff can be an important step in their healing.

CASE CONCLUSION

The parents are allowed in the room during the pronouncement. After death is pronounced, the attending and the nurses turn to the parents to discuss next steps. Because of the nature of the case described here, the deceased child becomes the custody of local investigating authorities; thus, all care post pronouncement needs approval. The nurses ensure that the infant has the IV lines removed, but they do not remove the endotracheal tube. Per local medical examiner guidelines, the nurse remains present with the parents. The parents stay with the child for about an hour before they state they are ready to leave. Using their smart phones, they take a photo and per medical examiner guidelines they can take a handprint with a kit provided by the ED as well as a small lock of hair cut by the nurse. They are also provided with a list of bereavement resources in their community by the ED social worker. Once the parents leave, there is a 10- to 15-minute debriefing of the team caring for the child led by the charge nurse with all team members present.

ACKNOWLEDGMENTS

The authors would like to acknowledge the contributions of Laura Gould Crandall, Founding Member and President of the Sudden Unexplained Death in Childhood (SUDC) Foundation, to this chapter, who in 1997 lost her first child, Maria, to SUDC at the age of 15 months.

KEY POINTS

- Know and use the name of the child when speaking to the family.
- Parents who lose a child are at high risk for complicated bereavement.

- Opportunities for legacy making and life celebration don't require sophisticated interventions and should be optimized as permitted by the local investigating authorities.
- Provide verbal and written contact information for the involved medical examiner or coroner who will assume custody of the decedent.
- Postmortem coordination of care with primary care physicians and other specialists and follow-up with parents minimize trauma in medical providers and family.

Further Reading

1. Haas EA. Sudden unexplained death in childhood: An overview. In: Duncan JR, Byard RW, eds. *SIDS Sudden Infant and Early Childhood Death: The Past, the Present and the Future.* University of Adelaide Press; 2018: Chapter 3:65–85. https://www.ncbi.nlm.nih.gov/books/NBK513391/

2. O'Connell KJ et al. Family presence during pediatric trauma team activation: An assessment of a structured program. *Pediatrics.* 2007;120(3):e565–e574.

3. Tinsley C et al. Experience of families during cardiopulmonary resuscitation in a pediatric intensive care unit. *Pediatrics.* 2008;122(4):e799–e804.

4. Davies R. Mothers' stories of loss: Their need to be with their dying child and their child's body after death. *Journal of Child Health Care.* 2005;9(4):288–300.

5. Harrington C, Sprowl B. Family members' experiences with viewing in the wake of sudden death. *OMEGA-Journal of Death and Dying.* 2014;64(1):65–82.

6. O'Malley P, Barata I, Snow S. American Academy of Pediatrics Committee on Pediatric Emergency Medicine, American College of Emergency Physicians Pediatric Emergency Medicine Committee, and Emergency Nurses Association Committee on Pediatrics: Death of a child in the emergency department. *Pediatrics.* 2014;134(1):e20141246.

7. National Association of Medical Examiners Panel on Sudden Unexpected Death in Pediatrics. *Unexplained Pediatric Deaths: Investigation, Certification, and Family Needs.* Bundock E, Corey T, eds. Academic Forensic Pathology International; 2019.

8. Conners P. American Academy of Pediatrics Committee on Pediatric Emergency Medicine, and Emergency Nurses Association Pediatric Committee. Death of a child in the emergency department. *Pediatrics.* 2014;134(1):198.

9. Foster TL et al. National survey of children's hospitals on legacy-making activities. *Journal of Palliative Medicine.* 2015;15(5):573–578.

10. Jackson BL. Bereavement in the pediatric emergency department: Caring for those who care for others. *Pediatric Nursing.* 2017;43(3):113–119.

11. Janzen L, Cadell S, Westhues A. From death notification through the funeral: Bereaved parents' experiences and their advice to professionals. *Omega-Journal of Death and Dying.* 2004;48(2):149–164.

12. Knapp J, Mulligan-Smith D. Death of a child in the emergency department. *Pediatrics.* 2005;115(5):1432–1437.

13. Merchant SJ et al. Exploring the psychological effects of deceased organ donation on the families of the organ donors. *Clinical Transplantation.* 2008;22(3):341–347.

14. Shoenberger JM et al. Death notification in the emergency department: Survivors and physicians. *The Western Journal of Emergency Medicine.* 2013;14(2):181–185. doi:10.5811/westjem.2012.10.14193.

15. Kenyon BL. Current research in children's conceptions of death: A critical review. *OMEGA-Journal of Death and Dying.* 2014;43(1):63–91.

16. Treadway K. The code. *N Engl J Med.* 2007;357(13):1273–1275.

14 Let's Get It Right

Sangeeta Lamba and Rebecca Goett

Case: An 88-year-old female nursing home resident with advanced dementia (bed bound and requiring full assistance for all activities of daily living) presents to the emergency department (ED) for altered mental status. In the ED, her vital signs are as follows: temperature of 38.2 °C, blood pressure of 90/55, heart rate of 125, respiratory rate of 24, and oxygen saturation of 92% on room air. Her chest X-ray reveals a right lower lobe infiltrate. Her daughter reports that over the last week she has been choking on thickened liquids and over the last 24 hours has developed fever along with increasing somnolence. Her daughter, who is her surrogate decision maker, also states that this is the patient's third visit for aspiration and pneumonia this year, and she wants her mother to be comfortable.

What do you do now?

HOSPICE REFERRAL FROM THE EMERGENCY DEPARTMENT

Seriously ill patients at the end of life will often seek ED care for multidimensional symptom control or signs of clinical deterioration, such as weakness, pain, fever, altered mental status, or difficulty breathing. For some patients at end of life, when their goals of care are consistent with a focus on comfort care versus disease reversal, hospice care may be a suitable option for disposition planning.

In the United States, hospice care is a system of care available to patients with a significant life-limiting prognosis who desire comfort care. While transitions to hospice care from the ED can appear daunting, this is often feasible. Regardless of ultimate disposition, hospice-eligible ED patients require thoughtful transitions to assess, align, and safeguard their goals of care. Hospice care in the United States is defined by the Medicare Hospice Benefit. As defined by this benefit, patients are eligible for such care when an attending physician and the hospice physician certify them as terminally ill, with a medical prognosis of 6 months or less to live if the illness were to run its normal course. For patients without Medicare, the hospice benefit is standardized and is delivered the same to patients with Medicare, Medicaid, private insurance, or no insurance. In 2018, 1.55 million people eligible for Medicare received hospice care—30% of whom had a diagnosis of cancer followed by heart disease/stroke (27%) and dementia (16%)—the remainder with all other diagnoses. The average length of stay for Medicare patients enrolled in hospice in 2018 was 89.6 days, and the median length of service was 18 days. The reasons for short hospice lengths of stay are multifactorial and include patient, provider, and system-based factors. However, patients who receive hospice care are more likely to have an out of hospital death, with lower symptom burden, with their families reporting better end-of-life experiences. Under the Medicare Hospice Benefit structure, the family is also entitled to bereavement care for the year after the patient's death. Outside of the United States, patients may receive the type of service described by the Medicare Hospice Benefit, but the service may be called palliative care and occur all along the care trajectory, including death.

The Medicare Hospice Benefit provides for four levels of care: routine home care, general inpatient care, continuous home care, and inpatient respite care. Payment for each level covers all aspects of the patient's care related to their terminal illness, including all services delivered by the interdisciplinary team and medications, as well as medical equipment and supplies. Each of the four levels of care is reimbursed at a different level.

- *Routine home care* is the most common level of hospice care, and this type of care is provided wherever the patient calls "home"—it may therefore include a nursing home, personal care home, or assisted living facility.
- *General inpatient care (GIP)* is provided for pain control or other acute symptom management that cannot be effectively managed in any other setting. GIP can be provided in a Medicare-certified hospital, hospice inpatient facility, or nursing facility that has registered nursing available 24 hours a day to provide direct patient care. Increasingly, hospitals may have the ability to deliver GIP on designated or "float" beds in the hospital setting, in partnership with a hospice agency.
- *Continuous home care* is provided for a period of between 8 and 24 hours a day in order to manage pain and other acute or distressing medical symptoms. Continuous home care must be delivered predominately as nursing care and supplemented with caregiver and hospice aide service. The goal of continuous home care is to maintain the terminally ill patient at home during a pain or symptom crisis.
- *Inpatient respite care* is available to provide temporary relief to the patient's primary caregiver. Respite care can be provided in a hospital, hospice facility, or a long-term care facility that has sufficient and 24-hour presence of nursing personnel. Respite care is typically only offered for patients who are already admitted to hospice care, and this cannot be an initial admitting level of care. Use of the respite level of care does not require the patient to have a worsening clinical status or symptomatic issue.

ED case managers, social workers, and an inpatient palliative care team, if available, are valuable resources if there is a question determining patient eligibility for hospice care and in helping establish the goals of care. That said, ED referrals for hospice care do not require consultation with a palliative care consult service if the emergency clinician is comfortable making

TABLE 14.1 **Key Questions for the Emergency Clinician**

Be Prepared to Answer These Questions	Be Prepared to Ask These Questions
· What is the terminal illness? · Who will be the attending physician? (If there is no primary clinician willing to serve as attending, the medical director of the hospice will serve in that role.) · What equipment will be needed immediately (e.g., home oxygen)? · What level of care is needed? · Is there a caregiver at home? · What is the code status? (Patients cannot be denied hospice enrolment if "full code"; however, the hospice team will need to know if code status needs to be addressed further.)	· How soon can you make an intake visit? (This includes coming to the emergency department then or soon after discharge if the patient is stable for discharge.) · Can you provide for the specific care needs of this patient to include specific medications and support needed such as . . . ?

referrals and utilizing available resources. Many outside hospice agencies can be contacted directly by the ED provider. Case managers and social workers in the ED can also assist in being the primary contact with the hospice agencies that are available within the area. Furthermore, case managers can help facilitate direct ED-to-hospice discharges within a reasonable ED or observation unit length of stay. To make a successful referral to hospice, the ED providers will need the information outlined in Table 14.1. In most communities, patients can be enrolled in hospice within 24–48 hours, regardless of the day; however, if hospice cannot be arranged in a safe, timely manner, admission to an observation or inpatient unit is needed until a safe discharge plan can be arranged. Once hospice is arranged, it is best to reconnect and orient the patient, family, and staff to the patient's care plans both during sign-out or discharge and to document this in the electronic health record, including the name and contact number for the hospice agency.

1. *Assess Medicare Hospice Benefit eligibility.* The patient should have a prognosis that limits their life expectancy to 6 months or less if the disease were to run its expected course, and the patient's care

goals are compatible with hospice. A useful starting point is to ask yourself, "Would I be surprised if this patient died within the next 6 months?"

2. *Discuss hospice as a disposition plan with the patient's physician.* Contact the patient's personal physician or the physician managing the patient most closely (e.g., the internist, family physician, oncologist, cardiologist, or nephrologist) and discuss the ED presentation, the patient's current condition, prognosis, and prior goals-of-care conversations. If you are considering hospice care, ask if the physician is willing to be the following physician for hospice services.

3. *Assess whether the patient care goals are consistent with hospice care.* Generally, this means a patient wants medical treatments and other support focused on symptoms and maintaining quality of life without focusing on life-prolonging interventions. The clinician should address issues such as a desire for further evaluations, rehospitalization, and disease-directed intervention. While most patients who elect hospice care will also elect not to have intubation or resuscitation at end of life, the Medicare Hospice Benefit does not specifically require this.

4. *Introduce hospice to the patient and family/surrogates.* The ED clinician should be able to discuss with the patient and family what hospice care is and what it covers. They should also be able to discuss some of the core aspects of hospice care, such as 24/7 on-call assistance, home visits for symptom management, coordinated care with the patient's primary physician, emotional and chaplaincy support, and so on.

5. *Make a referral and write orders.* When making a referral to hospice care, the ED clinician should be prepared to *ask* key questions such as How soon can you make an intake visit? (e.g., coming to the ED then or soon after discharge if the patient is stable for discharge). The ED should ensure that the hospice agency can provide for the specific care needs of the patient to include specific medications and support needs. The emergency clinician should be prepared to *answer* these key questions: (1) What is the terminal illness?; (2) Who will be the attending physician? (If there is no primary

clinician willing to serve as attending, the medical director of the hospice will service in that role); (3) What equipment will be needed immediately (e.g., home oxygen)?; (4) What level of care is needed and is there a caregiver at home?; and (5) What is the code status? (Patients cannot be denied hospice enrollment if "full code"; however, the hospice team will need to know if code status needs to be addressed further).

Sometimes patients who are undecided may only be ready to accept an informational visit in their home at a later time, for example, from a hospice representative after emergency discharge or during their hospital admission. The emergency clinician therefore serves an important role as the catalyst to this ongoing conversation. Some patients may require a stay in the hospital to stabilize or optimize their acute presentation, and this would be followed by hospice as a discharge plan. While hospice evaluation is underway, the patient's distressing symptoms should be explored, addressed, and managed effectively. Thoughtful transitions to hospice care for ED patients may require considering dispositions beyond the traditional paradigm of admission versus discharge such as arranging quiet rooms for the imminently dying patient while hospice care is arranged, inpatient palliative care unit placement or referrals to hospice for home placement after discharge from the ED or the hospital.

CASE CONCLUSION

On assessment, the patient has labored breathing and is in acute distress. You administer one dose of intravenous morphine 1 mg for the dyspnea and initiate antibiotics. The patient appears more comfortable, and there is ease of dyspnea after about 30 minutes. The emergency clinician has a goals-of-care conversation with the family and explains the clinical prognosis related to frequent aspiration as well as the acute episode of aspiration pneumonia in the setting of advanced dementia. The daughter expresses that she wants her mother's suffering to end and requests her mother be made comfortable and have a natural death at the nursing home. She does not want intubation or resuscitation to be performed should her mother's clinical status decline further. She feels her mother's quality of life is poor and her mother would not want further treatments that are not comfort care focused. The emergency clinician speaks to the ED social worker about hospice care. Simultaneously, the nursing home attending physician is called and all agree that hospice care would be appropriate to meet the patient's care goals. The daughter agrees to hospice care provided at the nursing home. Hospice is called for a home hospice level of care admission in the nursing home with an admitting diagnosis of dementia. The hospice agency worker comes to the ED that night to meet with the daughter to sign consent for hospice care. The patient is discharged to the nursing home with a plan not to continue the intravenous line or antibiotics and to continue those medications that are related to symptom control.

KEY POINTS

- Recognize that hospice consults requested in the ED potentially change the patient's trajectory of care—possibly with a patient going home to hospice care from the ED or after a short-term stay to control distressing symptoms.
- Identify patients who may be best suited for hospice team referral and also identify the healthcare team members who could support and assist in the transition, such as the case manager, social worker, or chaplain for spiritual support.
- Continue to provide effective control of symptoms and comfort care to the patients while they wait for transfer to the next setting, to avoid giving the appearance of "abandoning care."
- Clear and effective communication within team members and to the transitioning team (e.g., hospice agency, admitting team, observation unit, clinic coordinator) safeguards patient and family wishes and allows for accomplishing of the set plans of action.

Further Reading

1. Lamba S, Quest TE, Weissman DE. Initiating a hospice referral from the emergency department #247. *J Palliat Med.* 2011 Dec;14(12):1346–1347.

2. Lamba S, Quest TE. Hospice care and the emergency department: Rules, regulations and referrals. *Ann Emerg Med.* 2011;57:282–290.
3. Lamba S, Quest TE, Weissman DE. Palliative care consultation in the emergency department #298. *J Palliat Med.* 2016 Jan;19(1):108–109.
4. National Hospice and Palliative Care Organization. NHPCO Facts and Figures. 2020.

15 Just Call 911

Marie-Carmelle Elie

Case: A 32-year-old male with glioblastoma multiforme presents to the emergency department (ED) with increasing confusion. His wife reports that they are currently receiving hospice care at home for the last 4 weeks after their neurooncologist reported that there were no more options for cancer-directed therapy, but she was concerned regarding his confusion. She did not call the hospice nurse before coming to the ED. On examination, he is lethargic and opens his eyes to voice only. In the ED, his vital signs are as follows: temperature of 36.6 °C, blood pressure of 125/75, heart rate of 95, respiratory rate of 20, and oxygen saturation of 95% on room air. Serum labs are ordered by the triage nurse. Laboratory analysis reveals serum sodium of 155 mEq/L, chloride of 98 mEq/L, potassium of 5.3 mEq/L, carbon dioxide of 15 mEq/L, BUN of 40 mg/dL, and creatinine of 3.5 mg/dL.

What do you do now?

PATIENTS RECEIVING HOSPICE CARE IN THE EMERGENCY DEPARTMENT

This young patient presents with a neurologic malignancy in its advanced stages that is no longer amenable to cancer-directed therapy. The presentation of confusion and lethargy is concerning for swelling from vasogenic edema, as this places him at risk for seizures and herniation. Moreover, he has multiple laboratory abnormalities which are consistent with metabolic derangements, including dehydration and acute kidney injury. This patient is critically ill and is at great risk of dying in the ED. His enrollment in a hospice program confirms he has a terminal prognosis of 6 months or less, so that death is an expected outcome. The anxiety or stress that is experienced as the disease progresses may trigger a visit to the ED and be accompanied by requests to perform interventions that are not focused on comfort or consistent with the hospice philosophy. What are the priorities and responsibilities of an emergency provider to a terminally ill patient already enrolled with a hospice program?

In the United States, the Medicare hospice benefit is considered an entitlement available to people eligible for Medicare, Medicaid, or private insurance with a prognosis of 6 months or less if the disease runs its usual course and the patient and his or her family are interested in focusing on palliative measures for the illness. For those patients without insurance, hospice agencies provide indigent care. The hospice interdisciplinary team assigned to each patient includes a physician or nurse practitioner, nurse, social worker, and chaplain who develop a care plan aimed at meeting the personalized needs of each patient and their caregiver. The objective is palliation through the use of medications, therapies, and other modalities directed at reducing the symptoms associated with the underlying illness, including pain, nausea, anxiety, delirium, or dyspnea. Among the services and therapies that are considered palliative and may be covered under the hospice benefit are home health services, nursing care, antibiotics, chemotherapy, radiation therapy, physical therapy, speech therapy, wound therapy, and outpatient procedures such as thoracentesis and paracentesis drainage catheters.

In addition, and not dissimilar to admission to an inpatient service in a traditional inpatient hospital, there are various levels of care available with the hospice benefit to align with the clinical needs of the patient or that of the caregiver. The four levels of care are residential home care, respite care, continuous care, or general inpatient care. Residential home care represents the most utilized level of care in the United States where care is delivered in the patient's home. Typically this involves one to two visits per week by a nurse or other clinical provider in the home and other members of the interdisciplinary care team. Respite care is inpatient care provided to patients for up to a 7-day period in order to allow caregivers to attend to personal events, which may include appointments, an out-of-town trip, or a vacation. Respite care allows loved ones and families who are burdened by the stress of providing care with a few days of rest. Respite is typically provided in a facility such as a hospice house (care center) or a nursing facility. Continuous care is intense care provided for at least an 8-hour continuous period by a nurse in the home. This is typically provided for patients who are symptomatic and require the frequent administration of medication and monitoring. General inpatient care is provided in an inpatient facility for patients who require management of acutely symptomatic symptoms. Similar to continuous care, frequent administration of medication and monitoring is anticipated; however, this care must be provided in a facility. In the event the patient no longer wishes to continue on the hospice service, they may revoke their benefit and opt for traditional medical care.

Patients enrolled in a hospice program may present to the ED for various reasons. It is important that the emergency provider does not assume that the hospice presentation in the ED implies a revocation or rejection of those services. In circumstances where the patient is enrolled under the hospice benefit, the hospice agency is responsible for both the plan of care and is financially responsible for incurring all the medical costs related to their terminal illness. Care that extends beyond the plan of care for the terminal illness may not be covered by the hospice benefit, leaving the patient financially responsible if admitted to the hospital without the hospice agency's authorization. Before seeking care that could be related to their hospice diagnosis, patients and families are told to call the hospice agency first. This may or may not occur. In some instances, the patient has called the hospice agency and the hospice agency has directed them to the ED for care that is needed but cannot be provided by the hospice provider. Common reasons that hospice patients present to the ED include lack of symptom control, an event that could not be addressed in the home (i.e., fall and fracture; uncontrolled bleeding), failed device (i.e., tracheostomy dislodged), or service failure by hospice agency to communicate or provide timely response.

It is important to recognize that psychosocial and spiritual conflicts may frequently play a role in visits where there appears to be a "change of heart." The progression of symptoms in the patient and the witnessed decline by a loved one may evoke emotional distress, fear, and guilt, prompting a visit to the ED. Visits to the ED are considered either related or unrelated to the terminal illness. As an example, a patient with metastatic breast cancer develops a urinary tract infection and is found to have an obstructed ureteral stone, for which she is admitted, and a urethral stent is placed. Because the urinary tract infection and ureteral stent were unrelated to her terminal diagnosis of breast cancer, the cost of the hospital admission and the ureteral stent is the patient's insurer's financial responsibility. Engaging palliative care consultants, social workers, and chaplain services may assist in exploring issues influencing an ED visit.

Key steps to managing the case include the following: (1) notify the staff as soon as possible; (2) determine the trigger for the ED visit; (3) treat distressing symptoms; (4) work to reach a decision regarding the use of life-sustaining treatments (e.g., intubation for respiratory failure), if deterioration is imminent and rapid, and conduct a focused discussion around goals of care in the ED; (5) assess for cultural/spiritual needs, if the patient is actively dying; assure privacy; and endeavor to identify if there are any preferred locations a patient can be safely transferred to die (e.g., back home; to a private hospital room); (6) limit or withhold laboratory tests/diagnostics until discussion with the patient's hospice care team; (7) base therapeutic modalities on patient-defined goals of care; (8) plan a disposition after discussion with hospice staff based on the patient's goals; and (9) notify the inpatient palliative care service if the patient is to be admitted to the hospital. (See Table 15.1.)

Generally, the clinical approach should be focused on symptom management with limited diagnostic testing and imaging (see Box 15.1) to address the patient's immediate needs while simultaneously contacting the hospice agency, confirming understanding of hospice care, and assessing the goals of care to include an assessment regarding the understanding of illness and prognosis. Goals-of-care discussions are of paramount importance among

TABLE 15.1
Symptom Based versus a Diagnostic/Invasive Approach to Hospice Patients in the Emergency Department

Presenting Symptom	Symptom-Based Approach	Diagnostic/Invasive Approach
Dyspnea/respiratory distress in congestive heart failure	Opioids, diuretics, oxygen +/– BiPAP	ECG, CXR, TTE, laboratories, including troponin, BNP, Lasix, nitroglycerin, aspirin, oxygen, BiPAP, +/– intubation, admission, cardiology consultation
Agitation in advanced dementia	Neuroleptics, benzodiazepines	CT scan, laboratories, Haldol, admission, neurology consultation
Fever and dysuria in metastatic cancer	Antipyretic, empiric PO antibiotics (if desired)	Laboratories, cultures, CT scan, antipyretic, IV antibiotics, IV fluids, admission
Nausea, distension, and abdominal pain from advanced pancreatic cancer	Opioids, antiemetics, +/– nasogastric tube, steroids, octreotide, comfort food	X-ray, CT scan, surgical consult, morphine, IVF, nasogastric tube, NPO, admission
Seizure in patient with breast cancer and metastases to the brain	Anticonvulsants, steroids	CT scan, neurosurgery/neurology consultation, EEG, anticonvulsants, dexamethasone
Chest pain and shortness of breath in a lung cancer patient	Opioids, duonebs, oxygen	ECG, CXR, laboratories including troponin, BNP, CT angiogram, aspirin, oxygen

ECG, electrocardiogram; CXR, chest x-ray; TTE, transesophageal echocardiogram; BNP, B-type natriuretic peptide; NPO, nothing per oral; EEG, electroencephalogram; BiPaP, bilevel positive airway pressure; CT, computer tomography.

* Note that most symptom-based approaches can be achieved as an outpatient in the patient's home or a hospice facility.

patients identified as hospice or appropriate for palliative care in the ED. These discussions may clarify misperceptions, increase patient and caregiver engagement, increase opportunities for emotional and spiritual support, and improve rapport and satisfaction with the care team. Moreover,

BOX 15.1   **Key Steps to Caring for Hospice Patients in the Emergency Department**

1. Notify hospice staff as soon as possible. Under the Medicare Hospice Benefit, hospice agencies are legally/financially responsible for the patient's plan of care and all medical costs related to the terminal illness.
2. Determine the trigger for the emergency department (ED) visit. Pay attention not only to distressing physical signs and symptoms but also emotional and psychosocial issues. Involve social services, chaplaincy, and palliative care consultative services early if needs are identified.
3. Treat distressing symptoms.
4. If deterioration is imminent and rapid decisions are needed regarding the use of life-sustaining treatments (e.g., intubation for respiratory failure), a focused discussion around goals of care must occur in the ED.
   - Determine the legal decision maker if available and review any completed advance directives.
   - Complete a rapid goals-of-care discussion.
   - Make recommendations. For example, "According to what you want for [the patient], I would/would not recommend . . ."
5. If the patient is actively dying, assess for cultural/spiritual needs; assure privacy and endeavor to identify if there are any preferred locations a patient can be safely transferred to die (e.g., back home; to a private hospital room).
6. Laboratory tests/diagnostics should be limited or withheld until discussion with the patient's hospice care team. Testing should be based on patient-defined goals of care. Generally, low burden, noninvasive methods that may reveal reversible pathology or clarify prognosis should be used first.
7. Therapeutic modalities should be based on patient-defined goals of care rather than automatic "ED indications" (e.g., antibiotics for pneumonia should only be used if they meet a patient or surrogate defined goal of care).
8. Disposition should be planned after discussion with hospice staff based on the patient's goals. Returning home or a direct admission to an inpatient hospice facility may be the best disposition rather than hospital admission. At times, hospices can arrange 24-hour professional support in the home for patients with difficult to manage symptoms who wish to remain home.

9. Notify the inpatient palliative care service if the patient is to be admitted to the hospital. Hospice agencies may revoke a patient's enrollment in hospice care if care goals have changed, or they may continue a patient under hospice care during an admission for palliation.

Source: https://www.mypcnow.org/fast-fact/emergency-department-management-of-hospice-patients/

in those who opt for hospice care, there is an opportunity to garner these benefits early, affording the terminal patient with increased quality of life in the months before death. After clarifying goals and developing a shared plan of care with the patient and the family, communicate with the hospice provider to define the next steps as soon as possible. While some hospice patients may require an observation or inpatient admission, most will be discharged to their home or transferred to a hospice inpatient facility to continue care.

CASE CONCLUSION

In this case, the patient presents with lethargy and confusion, which is concerning for vasogenic edema. Labs were drawn and sent by protocol by the bedside nurse. While labs are abnormal, his vital signs are stable and he is protecting his airway. Given his lack of capacity to make decisions, you confirm that his wife is his healthcare surrogate. Having reviewed his medical records, you engage the wife in a discussion regarding goals of care. You ask, "What is your understanding of your husband's health condition?" She endorses a history of glioblastoma multiforme in her husband and states that they were told that there were no further treatment options. She reports that 2 days ago they had returned from a weeklong road trip, and he seemed tired but was otherwise acting normally. Today she had difficulty waking him up, and he seemed increasingly confused as the day progressed, though he had not been drinking alcohol. They have two small children at home ages 2 and 5 years. You now explain that you believe the tumor has grown and that surrounding edema may be encroaching on critical parts of his brain. She appears surprised and becomes tearful, stating "How could this be happening so fast? He was only diagnosed a month ago." You respond, "This must come as a shock, so soon after the diagnosis." She agrees and states that their decision to enroll in hospice would help decrease the burden to provide care in their home. He has a do-not-resuscitate order. To gather values and assess goals, you ask, "What was most important to him and his family?" She responds that he wanted to spend as much time with his family at home mentally intact so that he can interact with his children. He did not want his children to see him when he declined in a comatose state. When he became lethargic at home, she called 911, instead of hospice, fearing that the children might return home from daycare to find their father in a coma. "Based on what you've shared, am I correct in understanding that your husband values and prioritizes his ability to interact with his family?" The wife confirms. You contact the hospice agency, and they state that for quality of life they can try to empirically administer steroids to see if the patient will improve. The wife consents to this plan, and hospice agrees to starting steroids with a dose of dexamethasone 20 mg IV x 1 and to observe him in the ED. Four hours later the patient becomes increasingly more alert, and he is discharged home with hospice, who will continue to evaluate and provide steroids with the hopes that the patient might be able to interact with his family for some, albeit likely short, period of time.

KEY POINTS

- Patients with a prognosis of 6 months or less if the disease runs its usual course and the goals of care are consistent with a focus on symptoms and quality of life are eligible to enroll onto hospice.
- Hospice patients may present to the ED for reassurance and second opinion by the emergency clinician.
- The construction of a meaningful recommendation for the patient enrolled in hospice requires an assessment, a goals-of-care conversation, and alignment with the values shared by the patient and caregivers.

- Coordination of care with the hospice agency is required in order to ensure that the treatment aligns with the assigned care plan for the terminal diagnosis.
- Addressing emotional grief helps to establish rapport, resolve conflict, and prepare for the cognitive task of strategizing next steps.

Further Reading

1. Chan GK. End-of-life and palliative care in the emergency department: A call for research, education, policy and improved practice in this frontier area. *J Emerg Nurs.* 2006;32(1):101–103.
2. Smith AK, Fisher J, Schonberg MA, et al. Am I doing the right thing? Provider perspectives on improving palliative care in the emergency department. *Ann Emerg Med.* 2009;54(1):86–93.
3. Reeves K. Hospice care in the emergency department. *J Emerg Nurs.* 2008;34(4):350–351.
4. Lamba S, Quest TE. Hospice care and the emergency department: Rules, regulations and referrals. *Ann Emerg Med.* 2011;57:282–290.
5. Baile WF, et al. SPIKES—A six-step protocol for delivering bad news: Application to the patient with cancer. *The Oncologist.* 2000;5(4):302–311.
6. Fried TR, Bradley EH, Towle VR, Allore H. Understanding the treatment preferences of seriously ill patients. *N Engl J Med.* 2002;346(14):1061–1066.
7. Quill TE, Abernethy AP. Generalist plus specialist palliative care—Creating a more sustainable model. *N Engl J Med.* 2013;368(13):1173–1175.
8. Shearer FM, Rogers IR, Monterosso L, Ross-Adjie G, Rogers JR. Understanding emergency department staff needs and perceptions in the provision of palliative care. *Em Med Australasia.* 2014;26(3):249–255.
9. Meo N, Hwang U, Morrison RS. Resident perceptions of palliative care training in the emergency department. *J Palliat Med.* 2011;14(5):548–555.
10. Lu A, Mohan D, Alexander SC, et al. The language of end-of-life decision making: A simulation study. *J Palliat Med.* 2015;18(9):740–746.
11. The SUPPORT principal investigators. A controlled trial to improve care for seriously ill hospitalized patients: The study to understand prognoses and preferences for outcomes and risks of treatments (SUPPORT). *JAMA.* 1995;274(20):1591–1598.

16 "God Help Us"

Liliana Viera-Ortiz and
Clariliz Munet-Colón

Case: A 78-year-old woman with breast cancer
and metastases to the brain previously treated
with whole-brain radiation presents with
altered mental status for the last 3 days. In the
emergency department (ED), she is found to
have worsening brain metastasis with several of
the lesions noted to be hemorrhagic with midline
shift. The patient has become progressively more
lethargic. A goals-of-care meeting is held, and
the family reports that they believe that a miracle
will occur and state that God works through the
doctors and nurses to perform the miracle. They
insist that she be intubated and resuscitated
so that God can continue to "work." There is a
large family present and though the patient is
married and has named her husband as durable
power of attorney for healthcare, they state that
her brothers and sisters must make medical
decisions for her because they were with her
"first."

What do you do now?

SPIRITUAL AND CULTURAL CONSIDERATIONS

The patient in this case is an elderly woman with advanced metastatic breast cancer who now presents with a serious complication that is affecting her mental state, deeming her incapable of making her own decisions. Clinically, she appears to be deteriorating rapidly, and a prompt decision regarding resuscitation and intubation must be made. A bedside conversation with her family revealed their hopes for a miracle. The family would rather continue aggressive care so God can continue to work. Even though we know the patient chose her husband as her representative to make medical decisions, we do not really know the patient's wishes. Also her brothers and sisters appear to be under the impression that they are more deserving of making the medical decisions probably because of their close family ties and similar religious and cultural upbringings.

This case exemplifies the spiritual and cultural dilemmas that arise in the acute setting of an ED. Many times the emergency clinician has to make fast-paced clinical decisions for patients that are at the end of their life while balancing family beliefs and expectations. This can create multiple nonclinical challenges at the patient's bedside. Often spiritual, existential, and cultural dilemmas are left on the back burner as it seems priority ought to be given to clinical care. Nevertheless, spiritual and cultural issues often hinder clinical decisions and must be addressed in order to move forward with patient care. Clinicians need to have the right communication and clinical skills in order to better guide families in deciding what is best for the patient based on the latter's wishes and values.

Conflict may arise between the medical team and the family regarding the use of what may be felt to be medically nonbeneficial measures at the end of life. Although sometimes frustrating and difficult, an open and respectful conversation can enable better understanding of patient and family wishes, prognosis, and care options, as well as the religious and cultural beliefs behind preference for life-sustaining measures. Patients and families who feel heard and respected by the clinicians may be more willing to continue in respectful dialogue with the care team, even when their goals of care differ.

Spirituality versus Religion

Although spirituality and religion are terms that are often used interchangeably, there are differences between the two. Both concepts coexist and, more importantly, have been proven to be an integral part of a patient's experience during a life-threatening illness and end of life.

Most clinicians think it is appropriate to engage in discussion of spiritual issues when prompted by patients.[3] However, in general, they feel uncomfortable and unskilled to discuss religious and spiritual concerns (see Box 16.1). Reported barriers to addressing these issues include the lack of proper training and the perceived inadequacy of such training.[1] Lack of time and training are considered key barriers to spiritual assessment. According to findings from a national survey, over 90% of medical schools have courses on spirituality and health, but the content varies in scope and many times is offered as a single one-class lecture.[4] The lack of a solid educational foundation in spirituality and religion during the early years of medical education permeates to the graduate level, leaving residents and attending physicians equally unequipped and unprepared. Palliative care education can be an option for clinicians to better address these conversations.

BOX 16.1 **Spiritual Beliefs Conversation Starters**

- *Tell me more about the miracle you are hoping for.* This phrase is an open-ended statement we can use to learn more about the family's beliefs and religious views. This statement may enable us to learn more about how they define their miracle and hopes.
- *I see that faith is very important to you.* This is an empathetic statement that connects with their beliefs and can make them feel like the doctor is on their side regardless of his or her religious beliefs.
- *I also wish God can continue working through us.* "I wish" statements are useful to validate the family's faith and better align with their values without reinforcing something that may be improbable.

Source: Lo B, Ruston D, Kates LW, et al. Discussing religious and spiritual issues at the end of life: A practical guide for physicians. *JAMA*. 2002;287(6):749–754. doi:10.1001/jama.287.6.749.

Palliative care provides specialized medical care to patients who are experiencing severe illness, which includes holistic spiritual support. In the context of a life-threatening medical condition, patients seek for life significance and purpose as a mechanism to cope with an illness and its suffering.

At the Consensus Conference of Improving Spiritually in Palliative Care, *spirituality* was defined as the aspect of humanity that refers to the way individuals seek and express meaning and purpose, and the way they experience their connectedness to the moment, to self, to others, to nature, and to the significant or sacred.[7] Spirituality occurs within. It is an inner experience that one creates to connect personally with a higher power with hopes of finding a sense of peace and well-being.

Religion, on the other hand, refers to a communal dimension. It encompasses the set of dogmas and beliefs of a particular faith that belongs to a community of believers. It is the way the masses worship based on tradition, rituals, and scripture, and incorporate their beliefs into their ways of living. This concept can be intimately related to cultural beliefs, which we will consider further on.

Religious and spiritual beliefs equate the universe with God, which regardless of religion, could be defined as that Higher Being that is a source of comfort, peace, and hope. In the context of severe illness and nearing the end of life, many often see God and the "miracle" as the only way to achieve extraordinary healing when all medical interventions seem futile. Patients and families can also hope that God will continue "working" through doctors and nurses, and they may be seen as divine instruments as with the family from our case.[6] Many clinicians might instinctively dismiss the statement of a wish for a miraculous healing because chances for recovery are slim and supporting this belief may feel ill-advised. However, faith in miracles does not depend on their probability of occurrence.[5]

Conversely, important goals can be achieved by addressing and acknowledging their religious beliefs. First, clinicians have the opportunity to learn more about their own definition of the "miracle" and "works" of God. One can assume they are hoping for a cure or complete healing, but instead they may be hoping for more time with the patient, time to gather the family, or time to prepare for the imminent loss.

Second, clinicians should explore why continuing with aggressive life-sustaining care (intubation and resuscitation) may be part of their miracle.

This is the time where one can give clarifying information about the burdens of aggressive care in the context of advanced metastatic cancer and help them understand the patient's future. It may be appropriate to describe what the dying process might look like in a setting of aggressive resuscitative efforts and invite them to think about what the patient would have wanted if that were to happen. A helpful question one might ask the family to reflect upon could be: If the patient was able to participate in this conversation, what would he or she say in this situation? This question shifts the focus from what the family members want and centers it on the patient. Once the family understands the burdens of intubation and resuscitation, they might decide differently.

Lastly, acknowledging their beliefs may help create rapport with the family and open communication channels to better explore other treatment options like comfort care or hospice. Without this connection the family might feel unheard or dismissed, which could turn into disagreement and conflict.

Taking the above into consideration, let's examine some practical ways in which we can respond to the family in our case study. For possible responses, see Table 16.1.

TABLE 16.1 **Example Phrases to Explore Spiritual Beliefs**

What Not to Say	What to Say
"There's no time to talk about miracles right now. Let's talk about what you want done."	"Tell me more about her wishes."
"Most of the times miracles do not occur."	"I see that faith is important to you."
"Intubation will not prevent her death."	"I also wish God can continue to do His work."
"Her husband is the only person authorized to make medical decisions."	"I can see that she's important to you and you care a lot about her."

Source: Lo B, Ruston D, Kates LW, et al. Discussing religious and spiritual issues at the end of life: A practical guide for physicians. JAMA. 2002;287(6):749–754. doi:10.1001/jama.287.6.749.

A useful tool to elicit the patient's or family members' spiritual concerns is through the use of the FICA questionnaire, developed by Dr. Puchalski and her team.[8] It uses the acronym FICA: Faith, Importance, Community, and Address in Care. This questionnaire is meant to be integrated in the history of a clinical conversation in order to create an environment of trust and openness. The clinician can decide whether to mobilize additional sources of spiritual support like the hospital chaplain or clergy based on the patient and family's traditional beliefs. There are many known benefits to addressing the spiritual needs of our patients. It has been shown that patients who undergo less aggressive measures at end of life are more likely to develop feelings of realistic hope and less likely to die in the intensive care unit (ICU).

Culture

Culture includes the socioeconomic status, race, language, habits, traditions, and beliefs that define and give meaning to the members of a group.[2] Aspects of culture and their individual expressions may change through someone's life and specific circumstances. As a clinician, it is important to explore the patient's cultural beliefs and practices that influence medical treatments. Culturally appropriate care considers and integrates the patients and their families' cultural attitudes toward serious illness and death, their preference for care, and level of family involvement in the decision-making processes. Clinicians' failure to explore the impact of culture on how the patient and the family experience serious illness could limit respectful medical care. It may be helpful for clinicians to become familiar with commonly encountered practices and beliefs among different cultural groups without stereotyping or generalizing ethnicities. However, it is more important to humbly ask questions and be open to learn from the patient about his or her individual cultural background, a concept known as cultural humility.

Cultural Humility

The concept of cultural humility goes beyond memorizing cultural stereotypes or mastering the diversity of cultures. Practicing cultural humility means being open and willing to humbly explore the cultural background of patients and their families, and their view of serious illness, medical care preferences, and decision-making. It is a personal process where clinicians should, first, self-reflect on their own cultural stereotypes, prejudices, and unconscious bias that may be limiting the patient–clinician interaction. The concept of cultural humility implies understanding that being fully competent in a culture different from our own is seemingly impossible. Therefore, a way to learn about others is to identify our lack of knowledge with humility and ask them to share and explain their cultural practices and beliefs. Secondly, clinicians should explore the patient and family's values and beliefs that are guiding their medical decision-making process.

Figure 16.1 shows guided questions the clinician may use to further inquire about the patient's values and wishes for end of life. This humbling process of self-reflection and exploring the values and beliefs of the family

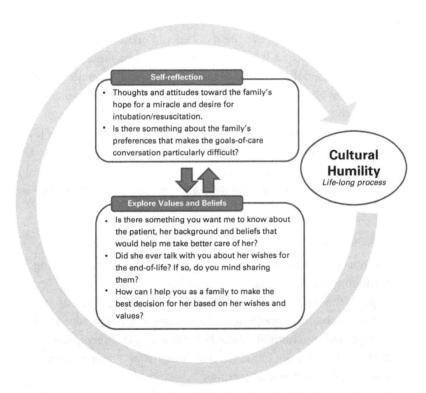

FIGURE 16.1. Practicing cultural humility: applied to the case. Guided questions to engage in self-reflection and awareness of unconscious bias and stereotypes and to explore the patient and family's values and beliefs.

helps to develop a closer relationship with the patient's family to engage in an open conversation to better discuss goals of care for the patient.

CASE CONCLUSION

The husband and her brothers and sisters insist on intubation and resuscitation despite the poor prognosis as they believe that God will perform a miracle through the doctors and nurses. The family relied on their faith as a way of keeping hope and emotional strength. Faced with this scenario, the clinician self-reflected about their attitude toward the patient's and family preferences. This self-reflection included the clinician asking themselves what their thoughts on the family's hope for a miracle were, and whether or not the family's requests are realistic. This family preferred to make decisions as a group rather than individually leaving the decision solely to the patient's husband. Even though spouses are the legal authorized decision makers by default and her husband is her legal representative by means of a durable power of attorney, the husband chose to include the extended family as they also know about the patient's values and wishes. After engaging in self-reflection, the clinician explored with the family these beliefs to learn more about the way they would like the medical team to care for the patient and determine a treatment plan (Figure 16.1).Based on discussions in the ED, the family opted to pursue hospice care. The emergency clinician was able to listen to the family and empathically acknowledge their spiritual beliefs.

KEY POINTS

- Connect by listening, acknowledging their emotions, and using sympathetic statements.
- Explore the patient's wishes and define "their" miracle.
- Include a chaplain, spiritual guide, or clergy in the patient's care.
- Practice cultural humility. Avoid stereotyping and recognize that personal biases influence our thoughts and actions with patients, families and colleagues.
- Learn the decision-making process of the family.
- Summarize and establish a plan with shared goals.

Further Reading

1. Balboni MJ, Sullivan A, Enzinger AC, et al. Nurse and physician barriers to spiritual care provision at the end of life. *J Pain Symptom Manage*. 2014;48(3):400–410. doi:10.1016/j.jpainsymman.2013.09.020.

2. Carey EC, Sadighian MJ, Koenig BA, Sudore R. In: Post TW, ed. *Cultural Aspects of Palliative Care*. 2022.

3. Curlin FA, Chin MH, Sellergen SA, et al. The Association of Physicians' religious characteristics with their attitudes and self-reported behaviors regarding religion and spirituality in the clinical encounter. *Med Care*. 2006;44:446–453. doi:10.1097/01.mlr.0000207434.12450.ef.

4. Koenig HG, Hooten EG, Lindsay-Calkins E, Meador K. Spirituality in medical school curricula: Findings from a national survey. *Int J Psychiatry Med*. 2010;40(4):391–398. doi:10.2190/PM.40.4.c.

5. Lo B, Ruston D, Kates LW, et al. Discussing religious and spiritual issues at the end of life: A practical guide for physicians. *JAMA*. 2002;287(6):749–754. doi:10.1001/jama.287.6.749.

6. Mansfield CJ, Mitchell J, King DE. The doctor as God's mechanic? Beliefs in the Southeastern United States. *Soc Sci Med*. 2002;54(3):399–409.

7. Puchalski C, Ferrell B, Virani R, et al. Improving the quality of spiritual care as a dimension of palliative care: The report of the consensus conference. *J Palliat Med*. 2009;12(10):885–904. doi:10.1089/jpm.2009.0142.

8. Puchalski C, Romer, AL. Taking a spiritual history allows clinicians to understand patients more fully. *J Palliat Med*. 2000;3(1):129–137.

9. Steinberg SM. Cultural and religious aspects of palliative care. *Int J Crit Illn Inj Sci*. 2011;1(2):154–156. doi:10.4103/2229-5151.84804.

10. Tervalon M, Murray-García J. Cultural humility versus cultural competence: A critical distinction in defining physician training outcomes in multicultural education. *J Health Care Poor Underserved*. 1998;9(2):117–125.

17 "Mine, No . . . Mine"

Jay M. Brenner

Case: An 89-year-old woman presents to the emergency department (ED) with respiratory distress and impending respiratory failure requiring endotracheal intubation. The ED clinician identifies that the patient has a healthcare proxy. The patient has two sons, both of whom share healthcare proxy. While there is an advance directive that names a healthcare proxy, there are no details regarding her wishes. The older son says that his mother would not have wanted to be intubated and is requesting withholding of life-sustaining treatment and a focus on comfort care. He says that his mother was explicit to him in her wishes not to have life-sustaining treatment. The younger son says that he wants his mother to receive life-sustaining treatment, including endotracheal intubation. He says that he cannot bear to lose her.

What do I do now?

SURROGATE CONFLICTS

Ideally, patients make their wishes clear about what interventions they would like, including cardiopulmonary resuscitation, endotracheal intubation, feeding tubes, antibiotics, intravenous fluids, operations, and procedures. Unfortunately, patients often lack decision-making capacity, and emergency clinicians must rely on surrogate decision makers to speak for the patients.

Classically, surrogate decision makers are expected to base this substituted judgment primarily on what they think the patient would have preferred if they were able to speak for themselves. Alternatively, they should base their representation on the patient's best interests if they do not know what the patient would have preferred. Experientially, in the setting where the patient has lost capacity, emergency clinicians may observe surrogate decision makers make decisions based on their own beliefs and interests and family consensus, perhaps with diminishing regard for the patient's wishes. Some contemporary ethics perspectives offer that surrogate decision makers base their practical decision on more surrogate-centered factors than patient-centered factors and that surrogates consider rather what their wishes are for themselves as a guide, reflect upon their religious and/or spiritual beliefs, their own best interests, a family consensus, and whichever decision helps them avoid guilt. While complex, clinicians must know their local statutes regarding who may ultimately serve as a healthcare decision maker. In jurisdictions where it is permitted, the emergency clinician may be allowed to align with a legally authorized individual(s) who offers the most convincing evidence of what the patient would have wanted if they could speak for themselves.

When time allows in the emergency setting, a best practice for managing surrogate conflicts is to have an urgent family meeting to elicit the patient's goals and values. While challenging in the emergency setting to have such a meeting, failure to do so might commit the patient to a clinical course that would not be in their best interest. In cases where action is required within minutes, the clinician may not be able to do more than identify that there is a conflict to be resolved later; the clinician must focus on actions consistent with what is legally binding, which most often will lean toward life-sustaining interventions until more can be known. When more time is available (e.g., a hemodynamically stable patient at end of life with days to weeks in the ED), involving many available perspectives is critically important. Optimally such meetings should be interdisciplinary and include the emergency clinician and nurse and possibly an ethics consultant or other independent mediator, such as a social worker.

NEGOTIATION WITH SURROGATES

Much like any clinical intervention, a family meeting may not succeed in resolving surrogate conflicts but ensures communication and the ability to assess the goals of care using empathic communication skills. Family meetings in the ED may take on various forms at the bedside and may be facilitated by audio or video conference call when persons cannot be present. While the surrogate decision makers, in this case, the healthcare proxies, may want more time to deliberate their decision, this may or may not be possible depending on the clinical status of the patient. Shifting the healthcare proxies discussion from what they would want to what the patient would want is the most important strategy in facilitating the meeting. The emergency clinician summarizes the clinical situation and informs the surrogate decision makers of the consequences of the intervention being recommended and the consequences of not doing it. In this case, endotracheal intubation may save the patient's life; however, it could also lead to prolonged suffering. Tapping into what the patient's values are may help this conversation progress. In addition to empathic communication skills, Table 17.1 summarizes some approaches that may be used in negotiations with surrogate decision makers.

In the setting where advance care planning documents exist with a particular perspective expressed, emergency clinicians may observe that a surrogate decision maker may represent a patient's wishes that do not seem congruent with previously documented wishes. This can be exacerbated when the advanced directive may be years old or does not seem to directly apply to the current clinical situation. While the clinician may experience moral distress, if they suspect the surrogate decision maker is advocating for what could conceivably be in the best interest of the patient based on a complexity of factors, proceeding with the surrogate's decisions can seem reasonable. While difficult to substantiate in the emergency setting, a healthcare proxy may harbor malicious intent. This may include expressing a wish

TABLE 17.1 **Approaches to Negotiation with Surrogates**

Technique	Notes
Build trust	Available to answer questions Engage someone who knows the patient (such as a primary care provider)
Educate and inform	Provide information regarding the patient's illness and prognosis
Provide more time*	Allow for more time for family discussions Suggest a time frame for rediscussion
Adjust roles	Remind surrogates that it's "the patient's decision" and encourage surrogates to remember it's a substitute decision Clinician provides recommendation based on goals and values
Highlight values	Reflection on the patient's values

*May need to proceed with interventions or treatments while more discussion is had.
Adapted from Brush DR, Brown CE, Alexander GC. Critical care physicians' approaches to negotiating with surrogate decision makers: a qualitative study. *Critical Care Medicine*. 2012 Apr;40(4):1080–1087.

to prolong a patient's life solely for financial gain or to induce more suffering upon the individual. Under these circumstances, unless there is clear and convincing evidence in the emergency setting, the emergency clinician should refer the case to legal and social services for further investigation.

EXPRESSED PREFERENCES VERSUS BEST INTERESTS

When a patient's expressed preferences are not clearly known, surrogate decision makers have to rely on what they think would be in the best interest of the patient. Some questions that Smith et al. suggest are as follows:

1. Is there time for deliberation? Is there a clear code status? In this case, the patient is in impending respiratory failure, and there is not much time for deliberation. There is also no clear code status order.
2. In view of the patient's values and goals, will the benefits of the intervention outweigh the burdens? This is the rub in this

case. Each son has a different interpretation. One son heavily weighs the value of survival of his mother, while the other son acknowledges the significant burdens of prolonged intubation and suffering.

3. Does the advance directive fit the situation? This question is not applicable in this case because there is no known advanced directive.

4. How much leeway did the patient provide the surrogate for overriding the advance directive? Unfortunately, this is not clear in this case.

5. How well does the surrogate represent the patient's best interests? This in the eye of the clinician. In this case, the emergency clinician hears one son saying that his mother would not want to be hooked up to a ventilator, because she had a significant decline in her quality of life since dancing at a family wedding last year. Meanwhile, the other son is thinking of his own loss if his mother were to die. It would seem that the former son would be representing his mother's best interests more so than the latter son's self-interest in avoiding his own grief.

AUTONOMY VERSUS AUTHENTICITY

Before resorting to best interests, Scheunemann et al. suggest asking these questions to ascertain a patient's values:

1. Was your loved one someone for whom it was important to live as long as possible, regardless of his quality of life?

2. What would your loved one think about her quality of life if it turned out that she would be permanently dependent on a mechanical ventilator?

3. What would your loved one think about his quality of life if he were unable to walk and had serious difficulty in doing daily activities like feeding himself or bathing?

4. How would your loved one think about her quality of life if she were severely cognitively disabled, in terms of having limited ability to think or communicate?

5. How would your loved one think about his quality of life if he were unable to make his own decisions?
6. How would your loved one think about her quality of life if she became unable to hold conversations or interact meaningfully with you?
7. How would your loved one think about his quality of life if he had to endure ongoing discomfort from pain, shortness of breath, thirst, or other symptoms?
8. Did your loved one have any religious beliefs that would guide her medical treatment?

Answers to these questions may guide the surrogate decision makers to an approximation of the patient's preferences. Additional useful approaches may help open and close a meeting. To initiate a discussion, an emergency clinician may ask the family members to simply talk about what kind of person their loved one is. And to close out a meeting, it may be helpful to give the surrogates "permission" to make the decision that it's clear they are trying to make but afraid to.

OTHER FACTORS TO CONSIDER

Independence with Activities of Daily Living
How independent is your mother? An emergency clinician may want to ask this question focusing on the dignity of the patient. One must be careful not to imply that physical dependence on others diminishes the value of life, even though it may lessen the quality of life. In this case, the one son who favored withholding intubation shared a video of his mother dancing at a family wedding the previous summer. Her mobility in the meantime, however, had declined to the point where she was no longer able to dance.

Frailty
Many geriatric patients, in particular, suffer from a dwindling quality of life where they encounter injuries and illnesses of frailty. This patient had fractured her hip several months prior, and while she was able to have a hip replacement surgery, she now had to use a walker.

Cognition

The sons did not report any dementia in their mother; however, she was currently delirious from her significant respiratory distress and likely hypercarbia. Baseline cognition certainly plays a role in surrogate decision makers' assessment of their loved one's quality of life.

Pain and Discomfort on a Daily Basis

How much does your mother suffer every day? This may or may not be a helpful line of questioning, depending on whether or not it is a factor.

Religion and Cultural Background

This is a critically important aspect of a patient's value system. While their religion or culture may not dictate their beliefs, it may very well inform them. Asking what faith, how important it is to them, and what community they belong to may help identify their preferences for life-sustaining treatment. This patient was Christian and active in her church, although she was unable to participate as much in her religious community's activities because of her frailty. Her belief in God was also relevant, in that she believed that God's will would be done with or without medical interventions. This belief was known by both her sons and helped to establish some common ground.

CASE CONCLUSION

Midway through deliberation with the two sons who both claimed to be healthcare proxies, the patient's brother arrived with his wife. The patient was placed on noninvasive mechanical ventilation to allow some time for conversation. The emergency clinician asked for the whole family to step into an empty examination room for a moment along with the patient's bedside nurse and chaplain to facilitate a conversation. To further build trust, the emergency clinician was able to reach the patient's primary care physician who joined the conversation by video call. The emergency clinician explained to the family that the patient if intubated might not be able to be extubated. Her primary care physician stated that the patient had always said she would want to be independent and when it was "her time" she would be at peace and wanted to die comfortably. The emergency clinician validated all the perspectives of each family member in an empathic manner. The surrogates' uncle was able to reinforce the values of the patient that she wanted to be independent. The chaplain was able to incorporate the patient's stated faith preferences regarding the afterlife to bring comfort to the family. The patient's brother pleaded with his nephew's conscience to consider what the patient would have wanted. The surrogate's uncle was skillful in his empathy, acknowledging the surrogate's suffering and grieving. After a few moments, the younger son acquiesced to his older brother's stated preference, admitting that his mother would not want to be dependent on machines. The family had reached consensus. The patient was not intubated and shortly after had a natural death with her family at her bedside.

KEY POINTS

- When surrogates are in conflict, maintain focus on the patient's ascertained values, optimally in the setting of a family meeting.
- Surrogate decision makers may base their decision on what they perceive to be the patient's best interests if they do not know what the patient would have wanted.
- Clinicians, when at all possible, should seek to support the family to make difficult decisions with as little guilt as possible using communication skills commonly employed in goals-of-care conversations.
- Clinicians that suspect malintent by the surrogate decision maker should enlist the help of the interdisciplinary team to include social workers and legal advisors.
- Clinicians should be familiar with their local statutes regarding who may ultimately serve as a healthcare decision maker while respectfully navigating conflict.

Further Reading

1. Kerckhoffs MC, Senekal J, van Dijk D, et al. Framework to support the process of decision-making on life-sustaining treatments in the ICU: Results of a Delphi study. *Crit Care Med.* 2020;48(5):645–653.

2. Mehter HM, McCannon JB, Clark JA, Wiener RS. Physician approaches to conflict with families surrounding end-of-life decision-making in the intensive care unit: A qualitative study. *Ann Am Thorac Soc.* 2018;15(2):241–249.

3. Bruce CR, Bibler T, Childress AM, Stephens AL, Pena AM, Allen NG. Navigating ethical conflicts between advance directives and surrogate decision-makers' interpretations of patient wishes. *Chest.* 2016;149(2):562–567.

4. Talebreza S, Widera E. Advance directives: Navigating conflicts between expressed wishes and best interests. *Am Fam Physician.* 2015;91(7):480–484.

5. Mickelsen RA, Bernstein DS, Marshall MF, Miles SH. The Barnes case: Taking difficult futility cases public. *J Law Med Ethics.* 2013;41(1):374–378.

6. Fritsch J, Petronio S, Helft PR, Torke AM. Making decisions for hospitalized older adults: Ethical factors considered by family surrogates. *J Clin Ethics.* 2013;24(2):125–134.

7. Scheunemann LP, Arnold RM, White DB. The facilitated values history: Helping surrogates make authentic decisions for incapacitated patients with advanced illness. *Am J Respir Crit Care Med.* 2012;186(6):480–486.

8. Brush DR, Brown CE, Alexander GC. Critical care physicians' approaches to negotiating with surrogate decision makers: A qualitative study. *Crit Care Med.* 2012;40(4):1080–1087.

9. Arras J. Ethical issues in emergency care. *Clin Geriatr Med.* 1993;9(3):655–664.

18 Global Aspect of Palliative Care

Emilee Flynn and Imad El Majzoub

Case: A 68-year-old woman with metastatic cervical cancer and a new spinal compression fracture presents to the emergency department (ED) in the city of Accra, Ghana, with severe, progressive back pain. She has been using paracetamol (acetaminophen) with only partial relief and asks if there is a stronger alternative available. She also reports increasing weakness and does not know if she can continue to care for herself. Her husband and children work daily, and she has no one to help her at home.

> **What is the best next step in the management of this patient?**

INTERNATIONAL ASPECTS OF PALLIATIVE CARE

There is an urgent and ever-growing need for the provision of palliative care services in all settings, especially in resource-limited settings. The World Health Organization (WHO), the World Palliative Care Alliance (WPCA), international working groups, national hospice, and palliative care associations, as well as other advisory organizations, have issued statements declaring palliative care an integral aspect of healthcare and a fundamental human right. Still, substantial disparities in access to palliative care services exist, particularly in resource-limited settings. In nearly one-third of countries worldwide, there is no access to palliative care services.

The Lancet Commission on Palliative Care and Pain Symptom Relief Study Group estimated that in 2015, 56.2 million people died worldwide. More than 80% of these global deaths occurred in low- and middle-income countries (LMICs), and as many as half of these individuals suffered from significant disease-related symptoms near the end of life, including pain, fatigue, weakness, dyspnea, anxiety, and depression. These individuals could have benefited from a palliative care approach at the end of life with a focus on reducing their symptom burden and responding to their suffering. Furthermore, it is estimated that an additional 35.5 million individuals experienced significant suffering secondary to nonfatal yet still life-limiting illnesses. These individuals can also benefit from a palliative care approach.

In children, defined in many international population studies as individuals ≤15 years old, the statistics are no better. The same Lancet Commission referenced above estimates that 2.5 million children died in 2015. Of the children experiencing significant suffering at the end of life, 98% lived in LMICs.

Experiencing constant pain can drastically impact patient outcomes, reducing both their satisfaction and their quality of life. Studies on the psychosocial effects of pain showed that patients with cancer repeatedly experienced higher incidences of depression and anxiety secondary to their pain. Prolonged pain can also impair concentration, making it difficult for patients to perform the basic activities of daily living. The patient described in the case above may be experiencing some of these effects, as she expressed her worry about her own ability to take care of herself in the future.

There are several factors that can help explain this disparity. In resource-limited settings, the ability to access quality healthcare remains scarce. Hospitals and healthcare centers are often located in more populated areas, meaning that individuals living in rural areas must travel great distances to reach care. Access to advanced diagnostic testing, even within large cities, may be limited. There are often too few trained and qualified healthcare professions. Those living in rural areas may turn to traditional healers who have different training and may provide alternative diagnoses and treatment recommendations for a patient's symptoms, further delaying the initiation of more evidence-based treatment strategies. All of these factors contribute to illnesses, especially oncologic conditions, being diagnosed at late stages thus further limiting the potential for curative therapies. Many of these patients with advanced disease will present to the ED for symptom management, as access to curative therapies and even consistent follow-up can be extremely limited.

The need to access high-quality palliative care services is far more pressing in resource-limited settings where diagnoses often occur in late stages of illness where curative therapies are limited and suffering is increased. And yet, as has previously been stated, nearly one-third of the world's population has no access to palliative care services. As can be seen with the provision of general healthcare within resource-limited settings, there is also a dearth of adequately trained healthcare professional capable of providing palliative care services and often no physical infrastructure in which to administer such care. The educational and training opportunities for healthcare professionals interested in palliative care remains limited, because much emphasis is placed on treating primarily infectious and communicable illnesses. In some settings there are different cultural and religious beliefs surrounding the utilization of certain medications and conversations about death and dying which may limit an individual's acceptance of hospice and palliative care services. There is insufficient access to medications to treat pain, especially opioid medications, and other symptoms—a topic which will be discussed in greater detail shortly. Many resource-limited settings lack comprehensive national plans which would help guide the development and integration of palliative care services. As healthcare systems continue to advance and begin to shift their focus from solely treating infectious diseases to adequately providing comprehensive care for noncommunicable diseases as well, there needs to be a concerted effort to ensure that palliative care is included within these national discussions and plans.

Efforts have been made to categorize the level of palliative care development within countries. Understanding a country's degree of development helps define opportunities for continued growth and identify areas where further and often intensive development efforts are still necessary. A six-part typology is used to describe the levels of development. As of 2011, the worldwide palliative care development efforts were described as follows:

- Group 1: No known hospice-palliative care activity, 75 countries (32%)
- Group 2: Capacity-building activity, 23 countries (10%)
- Group 3a: Isolated palliative care provision, 74 countries (31%)
- Group 3b: Generalized palliative care provision, 17 countries (7%)
- Group 4a: Preliminary integration into mainstream service provision, 25 countries (11%)
- Group 4b: Advanced integration into mainstream service provision, 20 countries (9%)

Figure 18.1 displays this level of palliative care development worldwide.

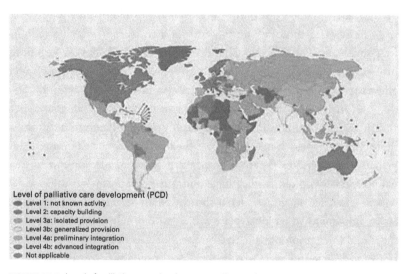

Level of palliative care development (PCD)
- Level 1: not known activity
- Level 2: capacity building
- Level 3a: isolated provision
- Level 3b: generalized provision
- Level 4a: preliminary integration
- Level 4b: advanced integration
- Not applicable

FIGURE 18.1. Level of palliative care development—all countries.

Understanding a country's degree of development helps to inform the interventions that can be recommended and provided to patients seeking care. Ghana falls into Group 3a: isolated palliative care provision. Despite the notable expansion of palliative care activism, it is still lacking harmony, unreliable, and not well coordinated or supported by national efforts. Funding for palliative care services remains largely dependent on private donations as such expenses are seldom included within national budgets. The majority of these services are offered in the home settings and reach only an extremely small percentage of individuals who need such services. Access to morphine, as well as other symptom management medications, remains exceedingly limited.

Opioid utilization is often used as a surrogate marker for a country's ability to provide palliative care services. Access to opioid medications remains remarkably inadequate in resource-limited settings, even in resource-limited settings where there is growing capacity for the provision of hospice and palliative care services. Morphine is considered an essential medication by the WHO and represents the top rung of the WHO three-step analgesic ladder. Yet despite these recommendations being in place for decades, more than 5 billion individuals worldwide have little or no access to essential analgesic opioid medications. Together, the United States, Canada, Australia, New Zealand, and serval European countries account for more than 90% of the world's opioid consumption. In contract, the continent of Africa has by far the lowest global consumption of opioid medications yet is the second most populated continent. Figure 18.2 depicts the distribution of opioid morphine equivalents worldwide. The image provides a striking contrast of the opioid utilization with a predominance of developed countries, including the United States, Canada, and Australia, and a near elimination of lower resourced countries, including those within both the continent of South America and the continent of Africa.

There are many barriers that contribute to an individual's inability to gain access to opioid medications in resource-limited settings. Opiophobia is often reported as the primary and most common reason for opioid refusal in resource-limited settings. Opiophobia is the fear of addiction and the fear of death when using this medication. The opioid epidemic that has gripped many well-resourced countries has contributed to this fear

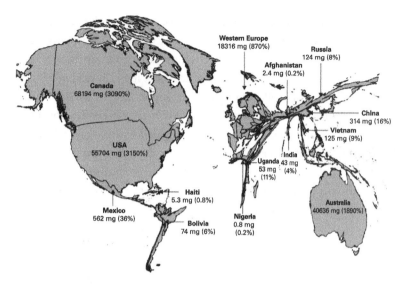

FIGURE 18.2. Distributed opioid-morphine equivalent (morphine in mg/patient in need of palliative care, 2010–2013), and estimated percentage of need that is met for the health conditions most associated with serious health-related suffering. This map represents countries by the size of their opioid consumption rather than geographical spread.

International Narcotics Control Board and WHO Global Health Estimates, 2015.

and further perpetuated many opioid myths. Healthcare professionals, policymakers, and patients fear that increasing availability of opioids, even in a controlled and monitored healthcare setting, will increase rates of addiction, misuse, and diversion to nonmedical use within the community As there is not current widespread use of opioid medications in resource-limited settings, the use of such medications is often reserved for individuals near the end of life. Consequently, many individuals correlate the use of opioid medications with impending death and refuse to take them, in fear that this means they, too, are dying. If they refuse this medication, there remains hope that additional treatment options are available. Many cultures also maintain the belief that individuals are expected to bear a certain degree of pain throughout their life. The inability to tolerate pain represents weakness. Additionally, without proper education, healthcare professionals may worry that the administration of opioid medications might hasten their patient's death. As the limited access to opioid medications is generally reserved for patients at the end of life, there is the false perception that such medications contribute to death, without the reasonable acknowledgment that it is in fact the severity of illness that has led to a patient's death.

Highly restrictive national government policies and regulations have further limited access to opioid medications. There are often burdensome licensing requirements that restrict which healthcare providers are able to prescribe opioid medications and which pharmacies can dispense such medications. Many countries require complex prescribing forms which can only be obtained from certain governmental offices. Pharmacies may be restricted to dispensing opioid medications only on certain days or at certain times in a given week. Consequently, many of these pharmacies choose not to stock opioid medications. Patients eligible to receive opioid medications may be limited to certain diagnoses regardless of symptom burden. The prescriptions these patients receive may only be valid for a limited number of days. There are often further regulations that restrict the amount of opioid medication that can be provided, permitting as few as 3 days of medication to be dispensed at one time. Individuals living in rural areas may be unable to afford transportation to and from clinics in cities to obtain and fill prescriptions for opioid medications. The price of the medication itself may be cost-prohibitive for many of these patients. Countries are less inclined to subsidize the cost of such medications given fears for addition and misuse and the perception that there are higher priorities deserving of this funding.

In settings where access to opioid medications is limited, healthcare providers should consider other symptom management medications. In the case above, the patient is only receiving paracetamol (acetaminophen), with partial relief of her pain. The addition of a nonsteroidal anti-inflammatory drug (NSAID) (e.g., ibuprofen) to the paracetamol can produce further analgesic effects. Even in settings where access to strong opioids is restricted, there may still be access to weak opioid medications, such as tramadol. Access to other adjuvant medications, including antidepressants, anticonvulsants, antispasmodics, bisphosphonates, and corticosteroids, should also be explored.

Similar to access to palliative care, the access to dedicated home hospice services is also severely inadequate in resource-limited settings. However, resource-limited settings most frequently possess robust and well-established community health worker (CHW) programs. CHWs are health workers who receive specialized trainings, often from local health centers or regional hospitals, but have not received formal nursing or medical training. CHWs are able to provide a wide range of services to the community, including basic health promotional, educational, and outreach services. They live in the areas where they work and are trusted and well-respected members of their communities. They frequently receive training to help identify common health conditions within their communities, including pneumonia, diarrheal illness, and malnutrition. This training allows them to identify conditions early, determine when certain conditions can continue to be treated in the community, and recognize worrisome signs that would warrant referral to the local health center or regional hospital.

In settings where access to palliative care is limited, programs have begun to explore training and utilizing CHWs to provide palliative care services. CHWs can raise awareness about the concept of palliative care in their communities, while concurrently identifying patients who may benefit from such services. They can provide education to the community about pain management strategies and help address myths and misconceptions that continue to exist about certain treatment options, especially around the use of opioid medications. They can also assist patients and their families by providing additional education about specific disease processes and increase both the patient's and family's ability to identify and monitor symptoms. They can also help to oversee procurement and administration of the appropriate pharmacological regimen where indicated. As members of the community with similar cultural beliefs and practices, they can provide additional psychosocial assessment and help to liaison with spiritual leaders in the community.

Established programs in India and throughout Africa have demonstrated that it is feasible to train and utilize CHWs to deliver palliative care services, particularly in rural and remote areas where the access otherwise remains woefully inadequate. Even in settings where access to opioid medication remains limited, CHWs trained in palliative care have been associated with reduced suffering of patients at the end of life. Training materials have been created which include both classroom training as well as clinical teaching through shadowing other healthcare providers already working in the field of palliative medicine. The concept of palliative care remained ambiguous in many communities, and CHWs were able to provide additional education about this field. They assisted in educating families in managing a patient's medical condition and symptoms and provided anticipatory guidance about the dying process. CHWs found that they were able to customize their practice, allowing for additional care targeting the growing emotional needs of patients and their families which often accompanies caring for loved ones at the end of life. They felt positively about their ability to provide comfort and support to patients and their families. CHWs primarily cared for patients who were incredibly ill. They shared with program evaluators that they could have benefited from additional training on caring for patients earlier in their disease trajectories as well as identifying and managing potential emergencies that can accompany the dying process. In general, CHWs reported a desire for longer training courses as well as the ability to partake in regular refresher courses and debriefing sessions with others providing similar care in the community.

CASE CONCLUSION

The case scenario at the start of this chapter describes a female patient known to have advanced cancer presenting with severe back pain to the ED in Accra, Ghana. The patient reports using paracetamol (acetaminophen), which did not adequately relieve her pain. The best next step in the management of this patient is focus on improving her current pain control. Given the limited access to opioid medications in Ghana, it is most reasonable to start by adding an NSAID. This addition is also supported by the WHO Three-Step Analgesic Ladder, where utilization of paracetamol and NSAIDs are the primary step in the ladder. Accordingly, ibuprofen was prescribed, and the patient was instructed to alternate administration of both medications, such that she receives either paracetamol or ibuprofen every 3–4 hours. She was also prescribed daily dexamethasone, a medication that is often readily available in the community as it has many indications for use. Anticonvulsants were considered; however, only patients with epilepsy can readily obtain these medications from trained mental health providers. (In many resource-limited countries, epilepsy is considered a mental health condition, and access to such anticonvulsants for indications other than seizures is restricted.) Antidepressants, antispasmodics, and bisphosphonates were also considered but were not available.

While there was no dedicated access to palliative care or home hospice services, the patient's village had an excellent CHW program. With the patient and her family's permission, she was connected with a trained CHW who lived in the same village. The CHW visited the patient frequently, which permitted her husband and children to continue working. This improved the patient's quality of life and led to an overall sense of relief as the CHW assisted the patient with several of her activities of daily living, thus reducing the burden on both the patient and her family. The patient's family members were able to continue working, knowing that the CHW would continue to care for their spouse and mother while they were at work. The CHW picked up the patient's medications from the pharmacy in the neighboring town and ensured that the patient was properly taking her medications, as per the schedule prescribed by the ED physician. Moreover, the CHW connected the patient and her family members with their community's spiritual leader, who provided additional counseling and support.

With the advancement of her disease, the patient continued to get weaker, was sleeping more throughout the day, and was eating and drinking very little. The CHW recognized these events as signs that the patient was approaching the end of her life. The CHW provided continuous emotional support for the family members and educated them about the dying process and remained with them until the patient died. As was their culture's accepted practice, the patient was buried in the village's cemetery the same day she died.

KEY POINTS

- Nearly one-third of the world's population has no access to palliative care services.
- 81% of individuals who experience significant suffering near the end of life die in LMICs.
- Barriers to adequate management of pain include limited access to opioids, opiophobia, lack of provider knowledge, national government policies, cost, and cultural norms.

In settings where access to strong opioids is limited, other analgesic medications, such as NSAIDs, weak opioids such as tramadol, and adjuvants, including antidepressants, anticonvulsants, antispasmodics, bisphosphonates, and corticosteroids, should also be considered. Trained CHWs can provide additional palliative care services, particularly in rural communities.

Further Reading

1. Knaul FM, Farmer PE, Krakauer EL, De Lima L, Bhadelia A, Jiang Kwete X, Arreola-Ornelas H, Gómez-Dantés O, Rodriguez NM, Alleyne GAO, Connor SR, Hunter DJ, Lohman D, Radbruch L, Del Rocío Sáenz Madrigal M, Atun R, Foley KM, Frenk J, Jamison DT, Rajagopal MR; Lancet Commission on Palliative Care and Pain Relief Study Group. Alleviating the access abyss in palliative care and pain relief-an imperative of universal health coverage: The Lancet Commission report. *Lancet*. 2018;391(10128):1391–1454. doi:10.1016/S0140-6736(17)32513-8. Erratum in: *Lancet*. 2018 March 9; PMID: 29032993.

2. Abu-Odah H, Molassiotis A, Liu J. Challenges on the provision of palliative care for patients with cancer in low- and middle-income countries: A systematic review of reviews. *BMC Palliat Care*. 2020;19(1):55. doi:10.1186/s12904-020-00558-5. PMID: 32321487; PMCID: PMC7178566.

3. Osman H, Shrestha S, Temin S, Ali ZV, Corvera RA, Ddungu HD, De Lima L, Del Pilar Estevez-Diz M, Ferris FD, Gafer N, Gupta HK, Horton S, Jacob G, Jia R, Lu FL, Mosoiu D, Puchalski C, Seigel C, Soyannwo O, Cleary JF. Palliative care in the global setting: ASCO resource-stratified practice guideline. *J Glob Oncol*. 2018;4:1–24. doi:10.1200/JGO.18.00026. PMID: 30085844; PMCID: PMC6223509.

4. Reville B, Foxwell AM. The global state of palliative care—Progress and challenges in cancer care. *Ann Palliat Med*. 2014;3(3):129–138. doi:10.3978/j.issn.2224-5820.2014.07.03. PMID: 25841689.

5. Lynch T, Connor S, Clark D. Mapping levels of palliative care development: A global update. *J Pain Symptom Manage*. 2013;45(6):1094–1106. doi:10.1016/j.jpainsymman.2012.05.011. PMID: 23017628.

6. Hannon B, Zimmermann C, Knaul FM, Powell RA, Mwangi-Powell FN, Rodin G. Provision of palliative care in low- and middle-income countries: Overcoming obstacles for effective treatment delivery. *J Clin Oncol*. 2016;34(1):62–68. doi:10.1200/JCO.2015.62.1615. PMID: 26578612.

7. Anderson RE, Grant L. What is the value of palliative care provision in low-resource settings? *BMJ Glob Health*. 2017;2(1):e000139. doi:10.1136/bmjgh-2016-000139. PMID: 28588999; PMCID: PMC5335766.

8. Berterame S, Erthal J, Thomas J, Fellner S, Vosse B, Clare P, Hao W, Johnson DT, Mohar A, Pavadia J, Samak AK, Sipp W, Sumyai V, Suryawati S, Toufiq J, Yans R, Mattick RP. Use of and barriers to access to opioid analgesics: A worldwide,

regional, and national study. *Lancet.* 2016;387(10028):1644–1656. doi:10.1016/S0140-6736(16)00161-6. PMID: 26852264.

9. Nchako E, Bussell S, Nesbeth C, Odoh C. Barriers to the availability and accessibility of controlled medicines for chronic pain in Africa. *Int Health.* 2018;10(2):71–77. doi:10.1093/inthealth/ihy002. Erratum in: *Int Health.* 2018 May 1;10(3):216. PMID: 29447356.

10. Hartwig K, Dean M, Hartwig K, Mmbando PZ, Sayed A, de Vries E. Where there is no morphine: The challenge and hope of palliative care delivery in Tanzania. *Afr J Prim Health Care Fam Med.* 2014;6(1):E1–8. doi:10.4102/phcfm.v6i1.549. PMID: 26245417; PMCID: PMC4502893.

11. Cleary J, Powell RA, Munene G, Mwangi-Powell FN, Luyirika E, Kiyange F, Merriman A, Scholten W, Radbruch L, Torode J, Cherny NI. Formulary availability and regulatory barriers to accessibility of opioids for cancer pain in Africa: A report from the Global Opioid Policy Initiative (GOPI). *Ann Oncol.* 2013;24(Suppl 11):xi14–23. doi:10.1093/annonc/mdt499. PMID: 24285225.

12. Saini S, Bhatnagar S. Cancer pain management in developing countries. *Indian J Palliat Care.* 2016;22(4):373–377. doi:10.4103/0973-1075.191742. PMID: 27803557; PMCID: PMC5072227.

13. MacRae MC, Fazal O, O'Donovan J. Community health workers in palliative care provision in low-income and middle-income countries: A systematic scoping review of the literature. *BMJ Glob Health.* 2020;5(5):e002368. doi:10.1136/bmjgh-2020-002368. PMID: 32457030; PMCID: PMC7252978.

14. Potts M, Cartmell KB, Nemeth LS, Qanungo S. A qualitative evaluation of a home-based palliative care program utilizing community health workers in India. *Indian J Palliat Care.* 2019;25(2):181–189. doi:10.4103/IJPC.IJPC_166_18. PMID: 31114101; PMCID: PMC6504743.

15. Yeager A, LaVigne AW, Rajvanshi A, Mahato B, Mohan R, Sharma R, Grover S. CanSupport: A model for home-based palliative care delivery in India. *Ann Palliat Med.* 2016;5(3):166–171. doi:10.21037/apm.2016.05.04. PMID: 27481319.

19 Caught in the Middle

Cynthia S. Romero and Lekshmi Kumar

Case: As a paramedic, you are called to the home
of a 59-year-old male with metastatic gastric
cancer under the care of home hospice with
increasing shortness of breath. On arrival he has
a temperature of 39.0 °C, heart rate of 130 beats
per minute, blood pressure of 70/30 mmHg,
a respiratory rate of 42 breaths per minute,
and an oxygen saturation of 82% on room air.
The hospice nurse has been called but has not
arrived. The patient has a do-not-resuscitate
order (DNR). His daughter is at the bedside
stating that he needs help.

What do you do now?

PREHOSPITAL PALLIATIVE CARE

Emergency medical services (EMS) arrive on scene to find a gentleman with respiratory distress and hemodynamic instability as evidenced by his tachypnea, hypoxia, tachycardia, and hypotension. Combined with fever and complaints of increasing shortness of breath in the setting of immunosuppression from metastatic gastric cancer, the patient meets criteria for possible septic shock from a likely pulmonary infectious source and has a higher mortality given the severity of his illness. EMS providers have a crucial role in this situation. They must not only discuss the goals of patient care with the patient and their family and hospice team but also provide rapid and appropriate care that aligns with the patient's end-of-life wishes and treat distressing symptoms. It is vital that they verify the patient's code status and other life-sustaining treatment orders early to help guide further management. In addition to the patient's clinical care, their responsibilities include explaining the critical condition, disease progression, and management to the patient's daughter, including the possibility of impending death.

The number of hospice and palliative care patients residing at home with life-threatening or terminal illnesses is steadily increasing as the population ages, with more patients dying in non-hospital settings.[1,2] This naturally translates to an increasing number of 911 calls for end-of-life emergencies.[3] Prehospital providers are often called on to assist in these situations and often feel ill-equipped, uncomfortable, and inadequately trained.[2,4] The primary duty of EMS personnel is often to save lives,[5] so management can be challenging when they are dispatched to an end-of-life emergency, where someone is dying and prolonging the patient's life may not be his or her main goal or desire.[1-4] It is imperative that EMS elicit the patient's plan of care before initiating treatment to ensure that patient's wishes are respected. In these situations, following established life-saving guideline may not be appropriate, and instead a different therapeutic approach that follows palliative care principles may be required, including "non-action" in order to allow patients to die with dignity.[5-7]

EMS providers must understand the key differences between hospice care and palliative care, so they are able to provide quality care to patients toward the end of their lives. Work by Connelly et al. identified knowledge deficits in EMS provider ability to correctly identify the nuances between "hospice" and "palliative care." Patients in hospice care in the United States require a diagnosis predictive of death within 6 months or less, if the disease runs its natural course.[5] Care focuses on reducing symptoms of their illness and improving quality of life, instead of undergoing treatments that are often futile or meant to prolong their lives. Most importantly, patients placed in hospice care are not required to have an active DNR order, which can often be an area of confusion for EMS personnel.[2] On the other hand, palliative care addresses physical, psychosocial, and spiritual care with the goal of improving the quality of life of patients and their families when facing a life-threatening, but not necessarily terminal illness. Palliative care can be initiated early on in an illness and continued through to death or cure of the illness, and often times includes therapies intended to prolong life.[8] Therefore, it is critical that EMS providers know that palliative care does not equal hospice care and being in hospice care does not automatically mean "do not resuscitate."

Hospice and palliative care patients and family members call 911 for a variety of reasons. Respiratory distress is the primary motive in most emergency palliative care calls. Additional reasons for emergency calls are neurologic complaints (coma or convulsions), uncontrolled pain, vomiting, pathologic fractures, massive bleeding, and panic disorder.[2,4,9–11] Although a patient's end-of-life wishes may be clearly documented, family members often feel uncertain about how to manage their loved one's symptoms at the end of their life.[3–5,7,12] Family members often feel terrified at the thought of their loved one's imminent death and, despite the patient's wishes, want to change the documented plan of care and have EMS do everything they can to "save" the patient.[3,10] Other times, patient's wishes are not documented, and when asked, family members must make hasty judgments as to what they believe is in the patient's best interests.[12] This situation is fraught with anxiety and high emotions as EMS personnel must balance respecting the patient's wishes and comforting family members.[3] Protocols established by hospice and palliative care teams to help patients and their families understand the dying process could potentially reduce the number of emergency calls toward the end of life.[3,5]

During these types of calls, EMS personnel must not only determine the presence of documentation regarding patient's end-of-life wishes but also the document's validity in an out-of-hospital setting as this guides their course of treatment.[2,4,7,13] Lack of documentation in situations where patients are dying creates uncertainty and variable decision-making by EMS personnel.[3] It can result in resuscitation initiation and/or transportation to an emergency department (ED), despite family expressing the patient's wishes to be otherwise.[13] Complicating matters is the variation in state laws regarding the ability of EMS personnel to make treatment decisions based on guidance from healthcare proxies, advance directives, and written medical orders.[7] Many states only honor advance directive and medical orders on state-approved DNR or physician/medical orders for life-sustaining treatment (POLST/MOLST) forms.[12] There is much confusion and misunderstanding regarding the differences between POLST/MOLST and other advance directives. The challenges with interpretation and using these forms by EMS personnel can negatively impact not only their ability to respect patient's end-of-life wishes but also patient safety and care for those who are transported to an ED for treatment.[11,14]

POLST or MOLST are a set of portable medical orders for patients with advanced, serious illness in a standardized format that focuses on critical care treatment decisions consistent with a patient's goals of management, used to inform providers especially when the patient cannot express their own wishes. Living wills are a type of advance directive where patients state their wishes about care and treatment they do or do not want, if they are no longer able to speak for themselves. Durable power of attorney for healthcare or healthcare proxy is a type of advance directive where a patient appoints someone else to make all medical treatment decisions for them if they are unable to themselves. An important factor to note is that in contrast to an advance directive, a POLST form involves the patient's physician in the execution process and requires a physician's signature. The POLST form can be utilized in all healthcare settings and can be acted upon by EMS in the prehospital setting. Another key difference is that a POLST form clearly outlines specific medical orders based on patient's wishes, whereas the advance directive only states the patient's wishes, which cannot always help guide management in the prehospital setting.[7]

There is also a difference between a DNR order and an out-of-hospital DNR order. A DNR order is a request to not have cardiopulmonary resuscitation (CPR) if the patient goes into cardiac arrest. While many patients have DNR orders completed while hospitalized due to the severity of an illness, this is not portable and does not equal an out-of-hospital DNR order. An out-of-hospital DNR must be signed by a physician for severely or terminally ill patients who do not want to be resuscitated at home or anywhere outside of a hospital facility. While some patients can wear bracelets or necklaces indicating their out-of-hospital DNR order, some state laws require a specific colored paper copy be visible or physically present before EMS can forego CPR. Therefore, EMS providers must not only be keenly aware of their state laws, but must be comfortable identifying these forms and understand what actions they can and cannot do during these highly emotional and stressful calls.

Equally important to EMS's comfort with these medico-legal documents is the human aspect of these emergency calls and how EMS cares for the patient's families. Education and training focused on interpersonal and communication skills so that EMS personnel can successfully manage conflict resolution and family emotions can improve preparation for these calls.[13] Waldrop et al. performed a study looking at prehospital providers' decision-making in end-of-life 911 calls and identified four decisional contexts depending on the family's awareness of the patient dying and documentation of wishes.[12] Even in the best of situations, when the family is aware their loved one is dying and the patient's wishes are clearly documented, EMS is called upon for comfort, professional presence, and for an explanation of what is happening. In situations where the family is unaware of the patient dying with or without documented wishes, EMS's role must transition to caring for the family by helping them move toward understanding the inevitability of death, consoling them, and helping them cope with the patient's sudden dying state.[12,13] In situations where a patient's wishes for DNR are documented, but the family becomes frantic and demands that orders be rescinded, EMS personnel must take into account scene safety and determine if a situation is becoming too volatile.[12] Such hostile environments may require EMS to load the patient and transport to the hospital for everyone's safety. Lastly, a major ethical conflict many EMS personnel encounter is the situation in which a family is aware of the dying process and patient's wishes for DNR are known, but those wishes are undocumented. Legally, without documentation being physically present, EMS must initiate resuscitation despite the fact that they know it is against the patient's wishes.[2,5,7,12] This creates an ethical conflict that often requires online medical control and may result in resuscitation with transport to the nearest appropriate facility. EMS providers can be better equipped to manage these types of situations with proper initial and ongoing education and training.

Research has shown that EMS providers require further training in the proper care of emergency end-of-life calls, with the quality of care depending on the expertise and knowledge of the EMS team.[1] While most EMS providers have cared for at least one hospice patient, studies have found that only 9.5% and 29% of prehospital emergency physicians and EMS providers have received any formal training in end-of-life care.[2,11] End-of-life care and advance directives are only briefly covered in the National Standard Curriculum for training of both emergency medical technicians (EMTs) and paramedics.[13] Multiple studies evaluating EMS provider comfort with end-of-life care have shown that most prehospital providers need and desire additional training and education, no matter how many years of experience they have in the field.[2,13] Lack of knowledge of medical information is a major problem in caring for hospice and palliative care patients in the prehospital setting. This is due to a variety of reasons, including locating critical end-of-life documentation, validating the legality of these documents, providing appropriate care that aligns with the patient's wishes, communicating with and comforting patient's families in highly emotional situations, and dealing with one's own emotional distress. These areas have been identified in various studies as being major areas of discomfort for EMS providers and suggests that EMS providers do not feel well-prepared to care for patients during end-of-life emergencies.[1,2,4,9,12,13] Research has shown that burnout, moral distress, and job dissatisfaction are common in providers caring for patients with life-threatening illness.[7] Current literature clearly shows that there is inadequate education and training that focuses on end-of-life emergencies in the prehospital setting worldwide, and thus represents the opportunity for systems improvement in prehospital end-of-life management. EMS personnel need to be trained on their local state laws and legal questions regarding the validity of medical orders and advance directives, interpersonal communication skills and empathy with patients and their families, and self-care for dealing with grief, emotional distress, and death. This will empower EMS providers with the skills and tools they need to successfully manage and provide quality care to this growing population of patients.

Collaborative networks between EMS and palliative care teams have demonstrated vast advantages, yet most of these studies have been completed outside of the United States in a Franco German model, where emergency physicians are often part of the prehospital team.[1,4,9] In one French study, collaboration between the prehospital emergency medical teams and palliative care networks allowed for better respect of the patient's care plan (83% of cases vs. 40% without collaboration) and avoided unnecessary transfers to hospitals (73% of patients transferred vs. 100% without collaboration).[9] While this study required significant planning and established guidelines for management of emergencies, it shows that through collaboration, the patient's wishes can be better respected and healthcare utilization can be reduced. Similarly, a prehospital German study found that EMS teams (including an emergency physician) with palliative care expertise sent significantly fewer patients to hospitals, instead treating more patients at home.[1] In contrast, in the United States, most EMS teams do not include an emergency physician being physically present; they are usually only available for online medical control. This can severely limit the ability of EMS teams to treat palliative care and hospice patients with analgesia, sedation, and anxiolytics without having to transport to the hospital if there is the lack of appropriate clinical care guidelines addressing their symptoms. The development of clinical care guidelines or treatment algorithms as guidance for all possible scenarios is challenging, as disease progression is often unpredictable. Guidelines that help EMS providers determine when to contact hospice or palliative care teams, and when and where to transport terminally ill patients can help with field decision-making by removing some of the uncertainty that arises with these types of calls.[13] Establishing prehospital protocols in conjunction with hospice and palliative care experts to address the most common complaints and symptoms seen in emergency calls for these patients may help EMS providers with their decision-making process.[5,7] A 2002 survey found that only 5.8% of responding EMS systems had a palliative care protocol;[5] while more systems may now have such protocols in place, it shows how widespread the conflict faced by EMS providers may be.

CASE CONCLUSION

In this vignette, EMS was called to the home of a 59-year-old male in hospice care with respiratory distress, hypoxia, and hemodynamic instability in the context of metastatic gastric cancer. The patient's hospice nurse has been alerted but has not arrived. EMS must clarify the patient's goals of care through discussions with the patient's daughter and hospice nurse (via telephone) and evaluate any advance directives, DNRs, and/or POLST/MOLST forms. This will subsequently help guide appropriate care and treatment of the patient, including symptomatic care such as intravenous fluids, analgesia, and oxygen for comfort. Lastly, and usually most difficult, is EMS's responsibility to help the patient's daughter cope with and understand that her loved one is dying. Ideally there should be specific protocols in place to help paramedics and EMTs manage commonly encountered symptoms in hospice and palliative care emergencies that are developed in collaboration between EMS, hospice care, and palliative care.

This vignette demonstrates how decisions made during end-of-life emergency calls can determine how and where patients die, whether the patient's autonomy is respected, and appropriate utilization of healthcare resources.[3] It highlights the importance of advance care planning in patients with terminal illness and toward the end of life, specifically discussing and documenting treatment wishes in the form of actionable medical orders, as well as educating family members about the dying process and what those orders mean for life-sustaining treatment. In the realm of prehospital care, treatment decisions usually depend on the presence of an out-of-hospital DNR or POLST/MOLST. Prehospital providers must feel comfortable not only understanding and interpreting medical orders and advance directives, but pronouncing death in the field, death disclosure, and comforting families in their time of greatest need. These facets of care require ongoing education and training for EMS providers, which will in turn significantly impact appropriate use of healthcare resources in this subsect of patients and result in respect for patient autonomy. It would be beneficial to integrate palliative care principles into EMS provider education not only from a healthcare expenditure perspective but also quality patient care perspective. Collaboration between EMS and hospice/palliative care networks need further development in addition to establishment and widespread use of prehospital palliative care protocols which can guide symptomatic care and treatment of hospice and palliative care patients during emergency calls in line with the patient's wishes. Synergistic collaborations between prehospital medicine, hospice care, and palliative care can have significant future implications that will benefit both patients and the healthcare system.

KEY POINTS

- Out-of-hospital hospice and palliative care emergency calls are becoming increasingly more common as the population ages and people live longer with chronic and life-threatening illnesses.
- EMS must elicit the patient's goals of care from family, the hospice team, and/or written medical orders before initiating treatment to ensure the patient's wishes are upheld and then provide timely care for distressing symptoms.
- When patients are dying, their families also become patients and usually require support, empathy, and comfort from EMS.
- EMS provider education and training in the emergency care of hospice and palliative care patients is severely lacking and should include the legality of and evaluation of advances directives and written medical orders, conflict resolution, communication skills, and coping skills for dealing with emotionally charged situations.
- Collaboration amongst EMS, hospice care, and palliative care is needed to create prehospital protocols for symptomatic care, comfort measures, and when transport to a hospital is indicated.

Further Reading
1. Wiese CH, Bartels UE, Marczynska K, et al. Quality of out of hospital palliative emergency care depends on the expertise of the emergency medical team—A prospective multicentre analysis. *Support Care Cancer.* 2009;17:1499–1506.
2. Donnelly CB, Armstrong KA, Perkins MM, et al. Emergency medical services provider experiences of hospice care. *Prehosp Emerg Care.* 2018;22(2):237–243.
3. Waldrop DP, Clemency B, Maguin E, Lindstrom H. Prehospital providers' perceptions of emergency calls near life's end. *Am J Hospice Palliat Med.* 2014;32(2):198–204.

4. Carron PN, Dami F, Diawara F, et al. Palliative care and prehospital emergency medicine: Analysis of a case series. *Medicine (Baltimore)*. 2014;93)25):e128.
5. Ausband SC, March JA, Brown LH. National prevalence of palliative care protocols in emergency medical services. *Prehosp Emerg Care*. 2002;6(1):36–41.
6. Duchateau FX. Palliative care and prehospital emergency medicine—Apparently conflicting approaches? *Eur J Emerg Med*. 2012;19(1):1.
7. Lamba S, Schmidt TA, Chan GK, et al. Integrating palliative care in the out-of-hospital setting: Four things to jump-start an EMS-palliative care initiative. *Prehosp Emerg Care*. 2013;17(4):511–520.
8. World Health Organization. WHO definition of palliative care. https://www.who.int/cancer/palliative/definition/en/. Accessed December 10, 2019.
9. Burnod A, Lenclud G, Richard-Hibon A, et al. Collaboration between prehospital emergency medical teams and palliative care networks allows a better respect of a patient's will. *Eur J Emerg Med*. 2012;19(1):46–47.
10. Rausch PG, Ramzy AI. Development of a palliative care protocol for emergency medical services. *Ann Emerg Med*. 1991;20(12):1383–1386.
11. Ferrand E, Marty J. Prehospital withholding and withdrawal of life-sustaining treatment. The French LATASAMU survey. *Intensive Care Med*. 2006;32:1498–1505.
12. Waldrop DP, McKinley JM, Dailey MW, et al. Decision-making in the moments before death: Challenges in prehospital care. *Prehosp Emerg Care*. 2019;23(3):356–363.
13. Waldrop DP, Clemency B, Maguin E, Lindstrom H. Preparation for frontline end-of-life care: Exploring the perspectives of paramedics and emergency medical technicians. *J Palliat Med*. 2014;17(3):338–341.
14. Jesus JE, Geiderman JM, Venkat A, ACEP Ethics Committee. Physician orders for life-sustaining treatment and emergency medicine: Ethical considerations, legal issues, and emergency trends. *Ann Emerg Med*. 2014;64(2):140–144.

20 From What to How

Audrey Tan and Danielle Stansky

Case: You are working in a community emergency department (ED) with 55,000 visits per year that is a regional referral center for oncology and heart and vascular disease. It has been identified that there are a number of patients who present to the ED who could benefit from symptom management, goals-of-care discussions, and referral for physical, spiritual, and psychological support. The ED director asks you to assist in the integration of palliative care in the ED. The hospital does have a hospital-based palliative care service.

What do you do now?

MODELS OF IMPLEMENTATION OF PALLIATIVE CARE IN THE EMERGENCY DEPARTMENT

Early palliative care integration is a topic that is becoming more important, widely discussed, and increasingly utilized in the ED. Fifty percent of Americans age 65 and older visit the ED in the last month of life. As a critical access point for the care of patients with advancing age and chronic serious illnesses, the ED is often the site of care for high-risk patients at a time of crisis, and a visit can often be an opportunity to address the patient's unmet palliative care needs.

There is a growing amount of compelling evidence for emergency medicine and palliative care integration with both improvements in patient-centered outcomes and a decrease in unnecessary healthcare utilization. The delivery of palliative care in the ED has demonstrated improvements in quality of life and symptom management. The initiation of conversations on advance care planning in the ED leads to increasing use of services such as hospice, which in turn leads to superior symptom management and improved caregiver bereavement outcomes. Impacts on resource utilization have also been examined. Palliative care in the ED leads to reduced inpatient admissions and decreases in hospital length of stays; furthermore, decreasing rates of 30-day readmission and intensive care unit utilization have been observed. As more research emerges demonstrating the benefits of palliative care in the ED, the demand for programmatic development and clinical solutions will only continue to increase.

Although there are clearly demonstrated benefits to integration, an optimal "one size fits all" model for a palliative care and ED integration has not been established. The challenges to standardization of a palliative care emergency medicine model include the vast differences in patient volumes, physical size, academic or nonacademic affiliation, acuity, and palliative care resources in EDs across the United States. Given these various considerations, a variety of models are offered as a framework for implementation, with the goal of curating the model selected to uniquely address each ED and institution's needs, targeted outcomes, available resources, and culture.

Based on the current evidence, there are three models for palliative care and ED integration:

1. Developing primary palliative care knowledge and skills for emergency providers
2. Facilitating consultation to a specialist palliative care service
3. Facilitating consultation to a dedicated palliative care team in the ED

Developing Primary Palliative Care Knowledge and Skills for Emergency Providers

"Primary palliative care" is the concept that all clinicians should possess the understanding and fundamental skills to address goals-of-care conversations and basic symptom management. Educational programs are focused primarily on providing emergency providers with the tools to address the palliative care needs of patients in the ED. Given the provision of palliative care is carried out directly by ED providers, this eliminates the reliance on specialized palliative care providers or additional staffing. The most significant barrier to this model is primarily related to the culture of emergency medicine. ED providers' acceptance of palliative care concepts and attitudes requires buy-in and a shift in existing ED culture. Thus, leadership support and palliative care champions embedded in the ED are critical to instill and reinforce the utilization of the palliative care skills and knowledge.

At a large academic tertiary care hospital in the New York metropolitan area, emergency providers were given training on initiating goals-of-care conversations in the ED, along with education regarding hospice services. Those patients with advanced illnesses and a prognosis of less than 6 months who presented to the ED subsequently received a goals-of-care conversation led by the emergency attending. If deemed appropriate, enrollment with hospice services was facilitated, leading to a significant increase in home hospice utilization.

Across the globe, a novel educational initiative developed at a large tertiary medical center in Taiwan was directed toward increasing emergency providers' comfort and knowledge in identifying and referring patients to hospice care. Emergency providers were given specific training on hospice and palliative care, rotated on the hospice unit, attended interdisciplinary meetings with hospice staff, and shared experiences between providers via a mobile communication program. This initiative led to a significant increase in hospice utilization and completion of advance directives for ED patients with advanced illness.

At a tertiary academic medical center in Singapore, patients who were actively dying or had a serious illness with a very high risk of mortality were managed according to a unique end-of-life pathway developed by an ED palliative care workgroup. The pathway consisted of a care bundle with clearly stated clinical management guidelines for emergency physicians and nurses, a private room, and initiatives for end-of-life care education for ED staff to facilitate the delivery of end-of-life care in the ED. The study proved the feasibility of a protocolized care bundle in assisting ED providers with the management of end-of-life patients.

More recently, a novel pragmatic study to test an intervention to shift the clinical paradigm of emergency medicine is underway. This four-pronged intervention focused on increasing primary palliative care skills and knowledge among emergency providers and consists of (1) evidence-based multidisciplinary primary palliative care education, (2) simulation-based workshops on communication in serious illness, (3) clinical decision support, and (4) provider audit and feedback. This intervention will be carried out at 33 different EDs over 2 years. Using Centers for Medicare and Medicaid Services (CMS) claims of beneficiaries in the patient cohort, outcomes analyzed will include healthcare utilization and survival following the index ED visit.

Facilitated Consultation to a Specialist Palliative Care Service

Programs that have a palliative care consultation team available at their institution may employ the traditional emergency medicine consultative model but incorporate novel workflows for rapidly identifying patients with unmet palliative care needs and expeditiously involving the specialty palliative care service. The benefit of these programs includes bypassing some of the known barriers to palliative care and emergency medicine integration, including the time constraints and busy environment often encountered by emergency providers. In this model, there is a well-established relationship between palliative care and the ED with novel triggers utilized to identify patients who may require a palliative care consultation in the ED. There may be dedicated personnel within the ED who screen patients, but ultimately, the consult is carried out by a palliative care specialist.

At an urban, academic ED, patients with known advanced cancer received an automated palliative care consultation, independent of emergency provider or oncology input, and had significantly higher quality of life at 12 weeks, although there were no differences in admission to the intensive care unit or hospice utilization.

At another busy urban academic medical center, a novel two-stage triage tool identified elderly patients with life-limiting conditions who were experiencing a decline in function, significant symptom burden, and high levels of caregiver burden from the ED. The tool was administered face to face by the project social worker. Emergency providers were subsequently notified of identified patients, and referrals to palliative care or hospice care were made by the ED team. Within an 8-month study period, 22% of ED patients older than 65 years were screened, and at its peak, this project accounted for half of the referrals to the palliative care service.

In a pilot study at an inner-city academic ED, emergency providers were asked to consult the palliative care team if an ED patient had an estimated prognosis of 6 months. Results show that within 6 months, emergency medicine providers identified 88 hospice-eligible patients with 91% accuracy. Fifty-seven percent of those seen by palliative care were discharged to hospice versus 30% of those not consulted. Patients were also enrolled earlier than the known institutional metrics, with a median hospice length of stay of 31.5 days.

Facilitating Consultation to a Dedicated Palliative Care Team in the Emergency Department

This model offers the highest level of integration, with the ED providing its own specialist palliative care services. The benefits of this model include circumventing the barriers traditionally encountered with involving specialty palliative care teams, who are typically only available Monday through Friday during business hours. Additionally, limited staffing on these teams often restricts their ability to be present in the ED emergently for palliative care consultation. These programs often possess unique efficient processes that are further developed to identify patients with palliative care needs such as workflows for expedited enrollment with a hospice or palliative care unit or case management of high-risk palliative care populations.

At an urban community teaching hospital, two palliative care nurse practitioners (NPs) rounded with the ED physicians and nurses to identify patients who may have palliative care needs. The NPs then delivered a two-step screening process to assess for physical, psychosocial, or advance care planning needs. If any needs were identified, the NPs would conduct a palliative care consultation. In a time period of 14 months, the NPs conducted 894 consultations with 10% of these consultations resulting in enrollment with hospice services.

Recently, a novel program dedicated to addressing palliative care needs in the ED was studied at an urban academic hospital. In this program, patients with active cancer in the ED underwent a five-question screen for unmet palliative and end-of-life care needs. Based on the results of this screen, an automated consult was placed to one or several existing ED resources, including a clinical pharmacist, a social worker, a transitional care nurse, or patient referral services. More than half of patients screened had one or more unmet palliative care needs and 30% received an ED-based palliative intervention with no impact on ED length of stay.

Implementation

An ED palliative care initiative starts with several critical steps to ensure successful implementation of a program to deliver high-quality and consistent care to patients and families with palliative care needs. The first and perhaps most important step is *developing a collaborative workgroup of ED and palliative care team members who are both interested and committed to the idea*. Given the initiative may have a broad impact, this group should include a range of individuals, including administrators and clinicians across multiple disciplines. These change agents or champions are critical to not only assisting in the development and implementation of the initiative but also in sustaining the change and the momentum of your program. The second step is to *complete a needs assessment to define the target outcomes and metrics for your initiative*. This step is critical to identify opportunities for improvement, justifies the investment in resources, and defines the targets that will be focused on. Given the local variations among EDs, it is critical to perform this assessment at the institutional level, focusing specifically on the unique profile of the ED in which the palliative care initiative is planned. Table 20.1 lists potential metrics to be measured.

The third step is *creating a reliable feedback mechanism to collect data to document program impact and to ensure that the initiative is achieving the desired goals*. One suggestion is to create an ED-palliative care dashboard to track the metrics and outcomes of interest, which can be developed at both an individual and departmental level. The fourth step is to *identify on-site and community hospice and palliative care resources that are available to the ED to assist in providing quality palliative care*. They can be grouped into four major categories, including clinical care, education, organization/utilization, and data collection/management. The final step is to *develop an action*

TABLE 20.1 **Potential Metrics To Be Measured**

Category	Potential Metrics To Be Measured
Operational	· Mean/median ED length of stay (hours) · Discharge status · % of 30-day readmissions · % of 30-day repeat ED visit · Number of hospice referrals · Number of palliative care referrals (if available) · Hospital direct cost (admissions only)
Clinical	· % of patients for whom the healthcare decision maker is documented in the medical record · % of patients with documented pain assessment on presentation · % of families with documented offer of spiritual support after ED death · % of patients in target population who have a documented palliative care assessment · % of caregivers in target population screened for caregiver strain
Patient satisfaction	· * of live ED discharged patients who reported that they were fully informed about their condition or treatment options · % of surrogates/families who report excellent end-of-life care after ED death · % of patients in target population reporting excellent pain and symptom management

plan. The key steps to developing the action plan include (1) establishing specific goals that address unmet palliative care needs; (2) setting project targets that are clear and feasible within a specified time frame; (3) identifying the changes in clinical practice and workflows required to achieve the targets; and (4) continually measuring progress in completing specific project goals through a system of follow-up and staff accountability.

CASE CONCLUSION

In this vignette, you meet with the director of the existing palliative care consultation service and based on local ED culture, volumes, palliative care team staffing, and administration's support, you together decide to implement a model in which ED consultations are facilitated to the specialist palliative care service.

You start by engaging a group of champions, which includes an ED attending with palliative care interest, a resident who had previously volunteered with a hospice agency, a nurse who is frustrated with the lack of palliative care in the ED, an ED social worker, a palliative care clinician who is interested in increasing engagement with the ED, and the ED administrator. During subsequent meetings, a needs assessment is performed, and the target population is determined to be oncology, vascular, and cardiology patients who may die within the next 6 months and require an expedited palliative care or social work consultation for a hospice referral to the local hospice agency. Clinical outcomes that are targeted include number of advance care planning notes documented while in the ED, change in pain assessment, and improvement in caregiver distress. Operational outcomes include increasing the number of palliative care consults and hospice referrals. It is decided that a screening question for high-risk patients will be completed by the ED clinician and ED nurse after they have assessed the patient, and either the nurse or clinician may initiate the consult to palliative care or the referral to hospice if appropriate. An ED palliative care dashboard is created to track the relevant outcomes.

During the initial steps of implementation, physicians, residents, physician assistants, and nursing are given education on palliative care concepts via online modules and during shift change by program champions. Contact information for the palliative care specialist team and the liaison for the local hospice agency is printed and posted throughout the ED. Outcomes of the initiative will be discussed at each faculty meeting.

KEY POINTS

- Each palliative care and ED implementation initiative will be based on ED needs and priorities, palliative care resources, and emergency provider attitudes and culture.
- Three broad categories for these models exist, but processes involved in each of the models may overlap and impact similar outcomes.
- Continual educational initiatives and a consistent palliative care presence in the ED will assist with achieving success in any palliative care initiative in the ED.

Further Reading

1. Wilson JG, English DP, Owyang CG, Chimelski EA, Grudzen CR, Wong HN, Aslakson RA; AAHPM Research Committee Writing Group. End-of-life care, palliative care consultation, and palliative care referral in the emergency department: A systematic review. *J Pain Symptom Manage.* 2020 Feb;59(2):372–383.

2. Grudzen CR, Stone SC, Morrison RS. The palliative care model for emergency department patients with advanced illness. *J Palliat Med.* 2011;14(8):945–950.

3. Hanning J, et al. Review article: Goals-of-care discussions for adult patients nearing end of life in emergency departments: A systematic review. *Emerg Med Australas.* 2019;31(4):525–532.

4. Wu FM, Newman JM, Lasher A, Brody AA. Effects of initiating palliative care consultation in the emergency department on inpatient length of stay. *J Palliat Med.* 2013;16(11):1362–1367.

5. May P, Garrido MM, Cassel JB, et al. Prospective cohort study of hospital palliative care teams for inpatients with advanced cancer: Earlier consultation is associated with larger cost-saving effect. *J Clin Oncol.* 2015;33(25):2745–2752.

6. Khandelwal N, Kross EK, Engelberg RA, Coe NB, Long AC, Curtis JR. Estimating the effect of palliative care interventions and advance care planning on ICU utilization: A systematic review. *Crit Care Med.* 2015;43(5):1102–1111.

7. Kelley AS, Deb P, Du Q, Aldridge Carlson MD, Morrison RS. Hospice enrollment saves money for Medicare and improves care quality across a number of different lengths-of-stay. *Health Aff (Millwood).* 2013;32(3):552–561.

8. Highet BH, Hsieh YH, Smith TJ. A pilot trial to increase hospice enrollment in an inner city, academic emergency department. *J Emerg Med*. 2016;51(2):106–113.

9. Huang YL, Alsaba N, Brookes G, Crilly J. Review article: End-of-life care for older people in the emergency department: A scoping review. *Emerg Med Australas*. 2020 Feb;32(1):7–19.

10. Shoenberger J, Lamba S, Goett R, et al. Development of hospice and palliative medicine knowledge and skills for emergency medicine residents: Using the Accreditation Council for Graduate Medical Education Milestone Framework. *AEM Educ Train*. 2018;2(2):130–145.

11. DeVader TE, Jeanmonod R. The effect of education in hospice and palliative care on emergency medicine residents' knowledge and referral patterns. *J Palliat Med*. 2012;15(5):510–515.

12. Smith AK, Fisher J, Schonberg MA, et al. Am I doing the right thing? Provider perspectives on improving palliative care in the emergency department. *Ann Emerg Med*. 2009;54(1):86–93.

13. Liberman T, Kozikowski A, Kwon N, Emmert B, Akerman M, Pekmezaris R. Identifying advanced illness patients in the emergency department and having goals-of-care discussions to assist with early hospice referral. *J Emerg Med*. 2018;54(2):191–197.

14. Weng TC, Yang YC, Chen PJ, et al. Implementing a novel model for hospice and palliative care in the emergency department: An experience from a tertiary medical center in Taiwan. *Medicine (Baltimore)*. 2017;96(19):e6943.

15. Grudzen CR, Brody AA, Chung FR, et al. Primary palliative care for emergency medicine (PRIM-ER): Protocol for a pragmatic, cluster-randomised, stepped wedge design to test the effectiveness of primary palliative care education, training and technical support for emergency medicine. *BMJ Open*. 2019;9(7):e030099.

16. Glajchen M, Lawson R, Homel P, Desandre P, Todd KH. A rapid two-stage screening protocol for palliative care in the emergency department: A quality improvement initiative. *J Pain Symptom Manage*. 2011;42(5):657–662.

17. Grudzen C, Richardson LD, Baumlin KM, et al. Redesigned geriatric emergency care may have helped reduce admissions of older adults to intensive care units. *Health Aff (Millwood)*. 2015;34(5):788–795.

18. Mahony SO, Blank A, Simpson J, et al. Preliminary report of a palliative care and case management project in an emergency department for chronically ill elderly patients. *J Urban Health*. 2008;85(3):443–451.

19. Reuter Q, Marshall A, Zaidi H, et al. Emergency department-based palliative interventions: A novel approach to palliative care in the emergency department. *J Palliat Med*. 2019;22(6):649–655.

20. Henson LA, Higginson IJ, Gao W, Build Care. What factors influence emergency department visits by patients with cancer at the end of life? Analysis of a 124,030 patient cohort. *Palliat Med*. 2018;32(2):426–438.

21. Gloss K. End of life care in emergency departments: A review of the literature. *Emerg Nurse*. 2017;25(2):29–38.

22. Lafond P, Chalayer E, Roussier M, Weber E, Lacoin-Reynaud Q, Tardy B. A hospice and palliative care bed dedicated to patients admitted to the emergency department for end-of-life care. *Am J Hosp Palliat Care*. 2016;33(4):403–406.

23. Chor WPD, Wong SYP, Ikbal M, Kuan WS, Chua MT, Pal RY. Initiating end-of-life care at the emergency department: An observational study. *Am J Hosp Palliat Care*. 2019;36(11):941–946.

24. Paterson BC, Duncan R, Conway R, Paterson FM, Napier P, Raitt M. Introduction of the Liverpool Care Pathway for end of life care to emergency medicine. *Emerg Med J*. 2009;26(11):777–779.

25. Ting SM, Li P, Lau FL, et al. Acute bereavement care in the emergency department: Does the professional-supported volunteers model work? *Eur J Emerg Med*. 1999;6(3):237–243.

26. Lamba S, DeSandre PL, Todd KH, Bryant EN, Chan GK, Grudzen CR, Weissman DE, Quest TE. Improving palliative care in emergency medicine board. Integration of palliative care into emergency medicine: The Improving Palliative Care in Emergency Medicine (IPAL-EM) collaboration. *J Emerg Med*. 2014;46(2):264–270.

27. Quest T, Herr S, Lamba S, Weissman D, IPAL-EM Advisory Board. Demonstrations of clinical initiatives to improve palliative care in the emergency department: A report from the IPAL-EM initiative. *Annals of Emergency Med*. 2013;61(6):661–667.

28. May P, et al. Cost analysis of a prospective multi-site cohort study of palliative care consultation teams for adults with advanced cancer: Where do cost-savings come from? *Palliat Med*. 2017;31(4):378–386.

29. Wang D, Creel-Bulos C. A systematic approach to comfort care transitions in the emergency department. *J Emerg Med*. 2019;56(3):267–274.

21 Not One More Thing

Carter Neugarten and David Wang

Case: You work in a large community hospital emergency department (ED) and feel that patients can benefit from palliative care consultation in or initiated from the ED. Several of your ED colleagues are unaware or unconvinced of the value of palliative care initiated from the ED, and ask that you substantiate the claim that palliative care consultation from the ED is useful. Why, when, and how should palliative care be consulted from the ED?

What do you do now?

THE WHY, WHEN, AND HOW OF PALLIATIVE CARE
CONSULTATION IN THE EMERGENCY DEPARTMENT

Why Should You Consult Palliative Care from the Emergency Department?

Patients with incurable, serious illnesses such as end-stage organ disease increasingly present to the ED with underrecognized palliative needs. These needs include functional debility, symptom burden, prognostic understanding, and caregiver burden.[1] More than 50% of geriatric and 80% of patients with metastatic cancer visit the ED in the final months of life.[2] These presentations often correlate with significant pivot points in patients' clinical and prognostic course.

Emergency physicians are uniquely positioned to recognize and take action on unmet palliative needs at these inflection points. ED-initiated palliative consultations have been shown to not only improve quality of life,[3] but also reduce downstream care utilization, leading to fewer ED revisits and hospitalizations.[4] ED-initiated consults significantly shorten hospital length of stay by an average of 4 days with fewer inpatient deaths.[5,6] Meaningful differences in clinical and financial outcomes result when palliative consultation is requested by the ED rather than per usual practice later in the hospital course.[7]

As health systems increasingly shift to value-based care, there is greater emphasis on financial stewardship without compromising quality of care. By proactively connecting eligible patients with early palliative care, emergency clinicians may align with their organization's priorities while enabling patients to receive treatment congruent with their goals of care.

Barriers to palliative care consultation include lack of understanding about palliative care, provider concerns, patient concerns, or familial concerns such as the idea that referral to palliative care make take away a patient's hope. While there may be internal tension for clinicians,[8,9] patients receiving palliative care have endorsed marked improvements in depression, anxiety, and well-being across multiple disease states.[10,11] In a brief ED visit, patients with serious illness can be introduced to the concept of palliative care and the continuum of palliative care to include outpatient palliative clinic, inpatient palliative consultation, or when appropriate, even discharge from the ED into a hospice program of care. While taking this extra step on a busy shift may seem burdensome, it is possible for an emergency clinician to make a significant difference in the care their patients will receive.

When Should You Consult Palliative Care from the Emergency Department?

It is a common misperception that palliative care is only appropriate at the end of life. More and more, patients are engaging with palliative care much earlier in their disease continuum, ideally at the time of diagnosis of a progressive, incurable illness and in partnership with their other specialists. Advance care planning discussions, especially delineation of medical power of attorney, gauging care preferences, and the acceptability of a "natural death," ideally occur in outpatient settings before approaching clinical extremis. However, due to numerous barriers, thorough discussions are often not held ahead of time, making the ED a unique location to initiate and continue these conversations. As the hospital gatekeepers, ED providers' conversations and decisions often commit patients to a clinical trajectory of care (e.g., intubation or intensive care unit [ICU] admission).

While clinicians might associate palliative care most often with advanced cancer, it is helpful to patients across a spectrum of disease etiologies. Palliative care plays an important role in the care of patients with illnesses such as advanced dementia, neurologic insults, congestive heart failure, advanced lung disease such as chronic obstructive pulmonary disease, liver failure, and renal failure.

There are many reasons to initiate palliative care consultation from the ED (see Table 21.1), though most consults pertain to managing complex symptoms or clarifying goals of care. The term "goals of care" encompasses much more than just code status. It also includes assessing patient perception of the serious illness, comparing acceptability of likely functional outcomes with quality-of-life tradeoffs, how loved ones are involved in caregiving and the decisional process, and how cultural or spiritual practices may shape medical decision-making. Even when it is not be possible for an emergency clinician to lead such an in-depth conversation themselves, the ability to recognize the need for and recruit palliative care to support potentially complex discussions in the ED can be critical.

TABLE 21.1 **Reasons to Initiate Palliative Consultation in the Emergency Department**

Unclear Disposition	Intended for Discharge	Intended for Admission
Clarify changes in choices for life sustaining therapies or ambiguous advance care planning documents	Symptom management to avoid hospitalization	Goals of care for anticipated patients with poor prognosis or continuity of care with existing palliative care relationship
Evaluating appropriateness of intermediary interventions in comfort care	Referral to outpatient/ home-based palliative services (warm hand-off)	Ethical dilemmas (e.g., surrogate conflict)
Currently receiving hospice care with unclear or changing goals	New enrolment on hospice	Complex symptom management (e.g., pain, nausea)

Adapted from Wang DH, Kuntz J, Aberger K, DeSandre P. Top ten tips palliative care clinicians should know about caring for patients in the emergency department. *Journal Palliat Med.* 2019;1597–1602.http://doi.org/10.1089/jpm.2019.0251

Palliative intervention may also significantly alter a patient's care trajectory. Acute illness and changes in clinical status heighten tensions for patients and families, and they can also be opportunities to realign goals of care. In these time-critical scenarios, early palliative consultation may result in avoiding ICU-level care, ED transition to comfort care, or direct discharge with the addition of hospice support. Palliative clinicians are also trained in hospice care, and they can provide guidance on how to best care for hospice patients in the ED or refer to hospice.

How Should You Consult Palliative Care from the Emergency Department?

When requesting palliative consultation in the ED, it is helpful to notify patients and caregivers that a palliative consultant will be seeing them. Doing so will improve the likelihood of a successful interaction. Family members often have false assumptions about palliative care, or after a quick internet search, think that it is synonymous with hospice care. Even a short introduction of what palliative care is by an ED clinician can improve the chance of a positive outcome. One brief way to describe palliative care is as an extra layer of support for patients with serious illness, with expertise in symptom management that can serve as a bridge between the patient and the rest of their care teams.

Initial inpatient palliative consults typically take an hour or more to perform, and palliative clinicians are not always familiar with ED workflows, time constraints, and the emphasis on disposition. As with any consultation, clarifying your consult question and urgency of request is helpful so that you receive the needed recommendations in a timely manner. When talking with a consultant, clarify if assistance is needed to help determine the need for admission (or level of care), if you are calling to obtain assistance with optimizing a discharge plan, or if the patient can be seen as an inpatient. Palliative care consultation may or may not lengthen ED length of stay. When palliative care consultation occurs after the patient leaves the ED, it still has been demonstrated to have tremendous value to and impact on patient care.

One strategy to communicate the urgency of the consult is as emergent, urgent, or standard. An example of an emergent consult includes a patient in severe respiratory distress requiring prompt intubation, though disagreement exists about the patient's wishes (e.g., they have a do-not-resuscitate order, but a family member is requesting intubation). Urgent consults include a severe malignant pain crisis that is not responding to traditional ED management. Standard consults are those that can take place as an inpatient within 24 hours. These include less acute symptom needs, or perhaps a patient with a tenuous respiratory status with COVID-19 who you think may decompensate and need intubation in the coming days, and there is lack of clarity about code status or goals of care. Other patients in which expediting inpatient consultation may be helpful include those with progressive illness such as organ failure or cancer, end-stage dementia, or patients with failure to thrive. Letting the consultant know that there are not immediate needs will help your consultants prioritize their workflow and provide appropriate support. This can be particularly helpful in EDs where patients board in the ED for long periods of time.

Palliative consult services may also have limited or no staff available in-house during nights and weekends, so it is important to establish

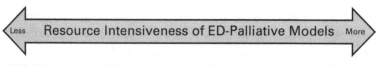

| PRN Palliative Consultation by usual ED practice | ED-triggers for Inpatient Palliative Consultation | Solo ED-embedded Palliative Clinician | Multidisciplinary ED-embedded Palliative team |

FIGURE 21.1. The spectrum of emergency department (ED)/palliative care partnership models.

beforehand expectations for unavailability during off-hours. Even if a palliative team is not available in person, they may still provide assistance in many other ways, including guidance over the phone, via video chat, seeing the patient the next day, or helping to facilitate a prompt clinic referral. In this way, palliative consultation from the ED may be helpful to both you and your patients in ways you may not have previously considered (Figure 21.1).

MODELS OF EMERGENCY DEPARTMENT/PALLIATIVE CARE CONSULTATION

The model of palliative care/ED partnership that your healthcare system adopts will depend on the needs, size, and resources of that particular system. Models can span a large spectrum, ranging from "as-needed" palliative consultation by usual ED practice, to dedicating and embedding a multidisciplinary palliative care team into the ED.

The least resource-intense model of palliative care consultation includes when the ED initiates as-needed consultation to an inpatient team per their usual workflows. This model may not lead to a significant number of consultations, but it can allow for ED/palliative care relationship development.

The next model incorporates standardized palliative care triggers into ED workflow to promote consultation. In this model, it is important to agree upon criteria that suit all stakeholders, taking caution not to overwhelm any party's workflows. Two examples of triggers that have been successfully implemented are the Palliative Care and Rapid Emergency Screening (P-CaRES) screening tool,[12] or a response of "no" to the surprise question: "Would you be surprised if your patient died in the next year?"[13,14] This "surprise question" has been validated in multiple disease states to help identify patients who would benefit from palliative care services.[15] The time frame used in the question can also be reduced from 1 year if there is concern of overwhelming a busy inpatient consult service.

Higher-resource models of ED–palliative care partnerships include embedding palliative care clinicians into the ED so that they can fully dedicate their time to seeing patients in the ED. Several institutions have implemented this model successfully, and typically a palliative clinician is based out of the ED during peak hours on certain days. Depending on staff availability and budget, this could be any member of the interdisciplinary team, including a physician, Advanced practice provider (APP), nurse, social worker, or chaplain. Sometimes, hospice organizations will also devote representatives to the ED to provide consultation and a potential link to hospice services.

The embedded clinician then actively screens patients in the ED for unmet palliative needs, is available for immediate consultation, and is more aware of ED time restraints and workflows. They can also screen for patients the palliative care team has seen in the past, thus improving continuity of care. The consultant can also develop relationships with ED staff, provide education and training on palliative care topics, and serve as a visible reminder of the assistance that palliative care consultation offers to ED patients, caregivers, and staff alike.

The fourth and final model would involve embedding a multidisciplinary team of palliative clinicians into the ED. For example, this could include dual ED/palliative care–trained physicians, APPs, EM-trained palliative fellows, and palliative-trained social workers. While this model would be the gold standard for ED/palliative care partnerships, it does not yet exist to our knowledge, and would be resource-intense and likely in need of further study and evaluation.

ED/palliative care partnerships often function best if there are "champions" on both the palliative and ED teams. This may include ED staff who are interested in palliative care and who remind the ED teams when consultation may be appropriate, or palliative clinicians with an interest in performing consults in the ED, including ED-trained palliative care physicians.

CASE CONCLUSION

In order to substantiate the claim that palliative care consultation from the ED is useful, your large community hospital changed the standard of care so that palliative care consultation was triggered for all patients whom the ED providers answered "no" to the surprise question, indicating a potential prognosis of under 1 year. Patients who received ED-initiated palliative care were found to have decreases in hospital length of stay and cost of 70% relative to standard palliative care consultation, consistent with the current literature.

Your hospital then approved the creation of new palliative care positions so that the ED could be staffed with dual-trained EM/palliative care physicians during peak hours, 7 days a week. After several months, this new partnership demonstrated value to the ED and healthcare system at large, and it is now a permanent fixture of ED care at your institution.

KEY POINTS

- Palliative care teams help care for many different patient populations and across many disease states (malignancy, organ failure, etc.). It is often best if they are involved early in the illness trajectory, starting at the time of diagnosis.
- There is a spectrum of models for how palliative care can support the ED, ranging from "as-needed" palliative consultation by standard ED practice, to dedicating and embedding a multidisciplinary palliative care team into the ED.
- Consultants can assist emergency clinicians with disposition (including direct ED to hospice discharges), decrease ICU admissions and readmissions, and shorten hospital length of stay.
- Palliative clinicians can also assist with difficult symptom management. Often, medication titration can be done safely and effectively in the ED and continued as an outpatient.
- When consulting palliative care from the ED, it is helpful to clarify your consult question, identify the urgency of your request, and notify patients that a specialist will be coming to evaluate them and provide an additional level of support.

Further Reading

1. Wang DH. Beyond code status: Palliative care begins in the emergency department. *Annals of Emerg Med*. 2017;69(4):437–443. doi:10.1016/j.annemergmed.2016.10.027.

2. Obermeyer ZCA, Makar M, Schuur JD, Cutler DM. Emergency care use and the Medicare hospice benefit for individuals with cancer with a poor prognosis. *J Am Geriatr Soc*. 2016;64(2):323–329.

3. Grudzen CR, Richardson LD, Johnson PN, et al. Emergency department–initiated palliative care in advanced cancer. *JAMA Oncology*. 2016;2(5):591. doi:10.1001/jamaoncol.2015.5252

4. Hui D et al. Impact of timing and setting of palliative care referral on quality of end-of-life care in cancer patients. *Cancer*. 2014;120(11):1743–1749.

5. Wu FM et al. Effects of initiating palliative care consultation in the emergency department on inpatient length of stay. *J Palliat Med*. 2013;16(11):1362–1367.

6. May P et al. Economics of palliative care for hospitalized adults with serious illness: A meta-analysis. *JAMA Intern Med*. 2018;178(6):820–829.

7. Wang DH, Heidt R. Emergency department admission triggers for palliative consultation may decrease length of stay and costs. *J Palliat Med*. 2021 Apr;24(4):554–560.

8. Allen LA et al. Anesthesia decision making in advanced heart failure: A scientific statement from the American Heart Association. *Circulation*. 2012;125:1928–1952

9. Ferrell BR, Temel JS, Temin S et al. Integration of palliative care into standard oncology care: American Society of Clinical Oncology Clinical Practice Guideline Update. *J Clin Oncol*. 2017;35:96–112. Babu D et al. Oncology providers' perceptions of early/concurrent palliative care. *J Pain and Symptom Mgmt*. 2016;51:421–422.

10. Bernacki R, Paladino J, Neville BA, Hutchings M, Kavanagh J, Geerse OP, Lakin J, Sanders JJ, Miller K, Lipsitz S, Gawande AA, Block SD. Effect of the serious illness care program in outpatient oncology: A cluster randomized clinical trial. *JAMA Intern Med*. 2019 Jun 1;179(6):751–759.

11. Sidebottom AC et al. Inpatient palliative care for patients with acute heart failure: Outcomes from a randomized trial. *J Palliat Med*. 2015;18(2):134–142.

12. Bowman J, George N, Barrett N, Anderson K, Dove-Maguire K, Baird J. Acceptability and reliability of a novel palliative care screening tool among emergency department providers. *Acad Emerg Med*. 2016;23(6):694–702. doi:10.1111/acem.12963. PMID: 26990541.

13. Haydar SA, Strout TD, Bond AG, Han PK. Prognostic value of a modified surprise question designed for use in the emergency department setting. *Clin Exp Emerg Med*. 2019;6:70–76.

14. Ouchi K et al. Feasibility testing of an emergency department screening tool to identify older adults appropriate for palliative care consultation. *J Palliat Med.* 2017;1:69–73.
15. Aaronson EL, George N, Ouchi K, et al. The surprise question can be used to identify heart failure patients in the emergency department who would benefit from palliative care. *J Pain Symptom Manag.* 2019;57:944–951.

Index

percutaneous endoscopic gastrostomy
(PEG) tubes, 104–5
performance status, 5
peripherally inserted central catheter
(PICC) lines, 102*t*, 105–6
pharmacokinetic considerations, 74
pharmacological measures, 52–54
benzodiazepines, 53–54
end-of-life care, 82*t*
nausea and vomiting, 60–52, 64*t*
for noisy secretions, 83*t*
opioids, 53
ventilator withdrawal, 127*t*
physiology, 51
PICC (peripherally inserted central
catheter) lines, 102*t*, 105–6
plan (REMAP tool), 8*t*, 31*t*, 33
policies, FWR, 116, 117*b*
POLST form (Physician Orders for Life-
Sustaining Treatment), 40*t*, 41, 42*f*,
85, 191–92
positive end-expiratory pressure (PEEP), 55
POST (Physician Orders for Scope of
Treatment), 40*t*, 41
posttraumatic stress disorder (PTSD), 114–15
PPS (Palliative Performance Scale), 5, 7*t*, 19
predictions for death, 19–20
pre-extubation simulation, 126
pregabalin, 95*t*
prehospital palliative care, 189–97
premedication regimens, 63–65
preparation, 28–29
Prescription Drug Monitoring Program
data, 94
primary palliative care, 1–11
case study, 1, 4–10
developing knowledge and skills for
emergency providers, 201–2
in emergency department, 2–4
overview, 2
Prognosis in Palliative Care Study Scores, 20
prognostication, 4–9, 13–24
case study, 13

challenges, 21–23, 30
communication in ED, 20–21
compatibility with hospice care, 142–43
time to death, 128
tools for, 19–20
trajectories, 13–19
prognostic awareness, 29–30
protocol, FWR, 116, 117*b*
psychological trauma, 114–15
psychology, 52
PTSD (posttraumatic stress disorder), 114–15
pulmonary rehabilitation, 52

quality of life, 23, 28, 190–91

radiation-induced nausea and vomiting
(RINV), 65
radiation therapy, 65
RDOS (Respiratory Distress Observation
Scale), 81, 124
recommendations, 9, 22*t*
based on values, 33
end-of-life care, 39, 46
referrals, hospice care, 139–45, 201–2
refractory CINV, 63–65
reframe (REMAP tool), 8*t*, 30, 31*t*
religion, 159–62, 173
REMAP tool, 8*t*, 30–33, 31*t*
renal failure, 74, 74*t*
rescue dose, 72–74
residential home care, 140–41, 148–49
RESPECT Project, 86*b*, 88
Respiratory Distress Observation Scale
(RDOS), 81, 124
respiratory distress or failure, 16–17, 81,
126, 191
respite care, 141, 148–49
resuscitation
family witnessed resuscitation (FWR),
109–19, 132–33
hospice care and, 143
procedures, 39
spirituality and, 160–61

RINV (radiation-induced nausea and vomiting), 65
rituals, 125*t*
room air, 54
routine (residential) home care, 140–41, 148–49

scopolamine (hyoscine hydrobromide), 82*t*, 83*t*
screening, 116, 216–17
secretion management, 83–84
self-care, 7*t*
self-reflection, 163*f*, 163–64
sepsis, 16–17
Serious Illness Conversation Guide, 20–21
serious illness conversations, 17–18
serotonin and norepinephrine reuptake inhibitors (SNRIs), 95*t*
serotonin antagonists, 62–63, 64*t*, 65
shared decision-making, 30
SIDS (sudden infant death syndrome), 132
Singapore, 202
somatic pain, 70, 92
somatostatin analogue, 64*t*
specialist palliative care service, 202–3
spirituality, 157–64
    considerations for, 158
    religion vs., 159–62
    supporting, 62–63, 124, 125*t*
standard consults, 215
steroids, 64*t*
subcutaneous infusion, 82
sudden illness trajectory, 14, 43
sudden infant death syndrome (SIDS), 132
sudden unexpected infant death (SUID), 132
sudden unexplained death in childhood (SUDC), 132
Sudden Unexplained Death in Childhood (SUDC) Foundation, 136
surprise question, 4–5, 19–20, 216–17
surrogates, 123, 125*t*, 167–74
    autonomy vs. authenticity, 171–72

conflicts with, 168–69
expressed preferences vs. best interests, 170–71
factors to consider, 172–73
negotiating with, 169–70
symptomatic loculations, 100
symptom control, 5
symptom management, 49–56
    aggressive symptom treatment, 82
    hospice presentation in ED, 150–53, 151*t*
    limited access to opioids and, 183
    nausea and vomiting, 60–62
    removal of LST, 125*t*

Taiwan, 201–2
TCAs (tricyclic antidepressants), 71, 95*t*
TDD (total daily dose), 72–74, 73*b*
terminal extubation, 122
terminal illness trajectory, 14–15, 43
terminal weaning process, 124
therapeutic modalities, 152*b*
Three-Step Analgesic Ladder (WHO), 181, 185
time-limited trial, 9, 33–34, 44–45, 46
time prognosis, 30
time to death, 128
time to maximal concentration (Tmax), 73*b*, 74
titration, 125*t*
tolerant, opioid, 71–72
tools, prognostication, 19–20
total daily dose (TDD), 72–74, 73*b*
total parenteral nutrition (TPN), 101
toxicity, opioid, 71
training, 116
trajectories, 5, 6*f*
    applying advance directives, 43–44
    palliative intervention altering, 214
    prognostication, 13–19
transplantation, 15
tricyclic antidepressants (TCAs), 71, 95*t*
triggers, 216–17